Yoga

for mother and baby

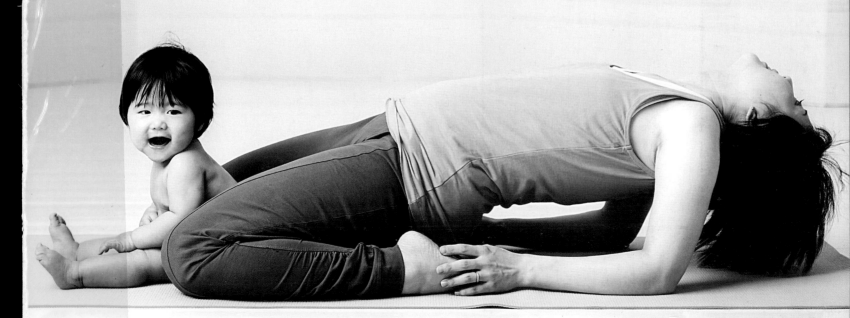

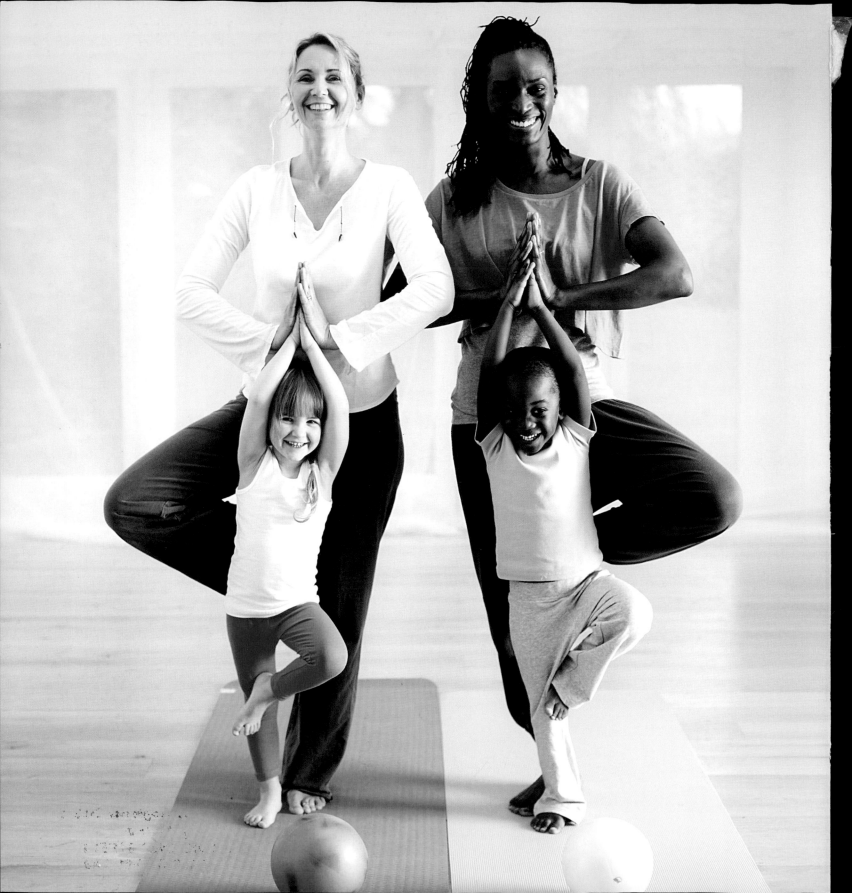

Yoga
for mother and baby

Interactive poses for you and your baby
(0–3 years old)

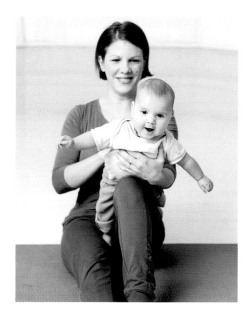

Françoise Barbira Freedman

in association with Birthlight Trust

CICO BOOKS
LONDON NEW YORK

Published in 2010 by CICO Books
An imprint of Ryland Peters & Small
20–21 Jockey's Fields
London
WC1R 4BW

519 Broadway, 5th Floor
New York
NY 10012

www.cicobooks.com

10 9 8 7 6 5 4 3 2 1

A CIP catalog record for ths book is
available from the Library of Congress
and the British Library.

ISBN 978-1-907030-61-1

Printed in China

Editor: Marion Paull
Designer: Jacqui Caulton
Photographer: Ian Boddy
Special Babies Consultant: Jay Ehrlich,
yoga therapist and special needs advisor
(www.yogababies.co.uk)

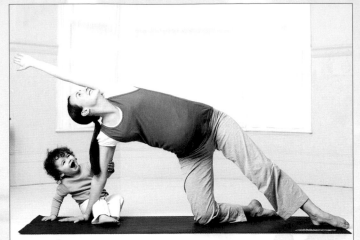

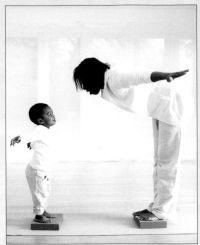

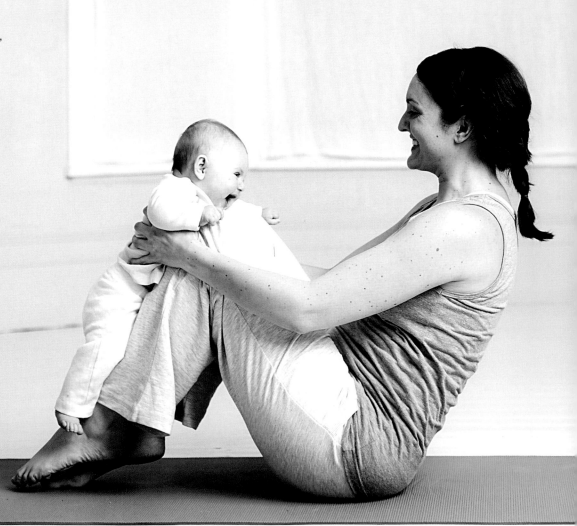

Contents

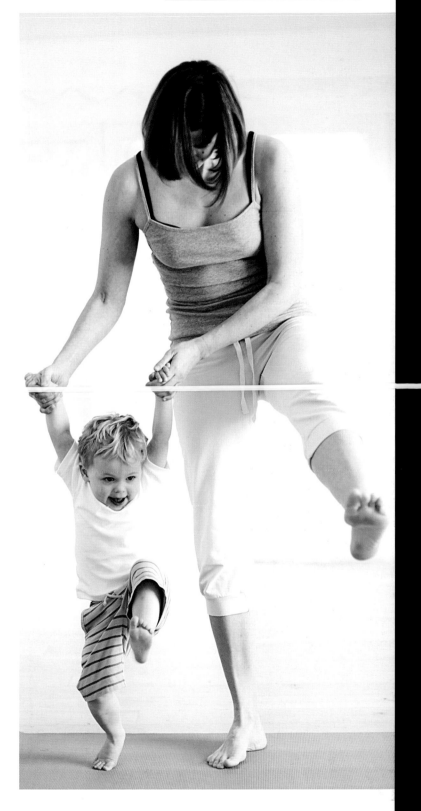

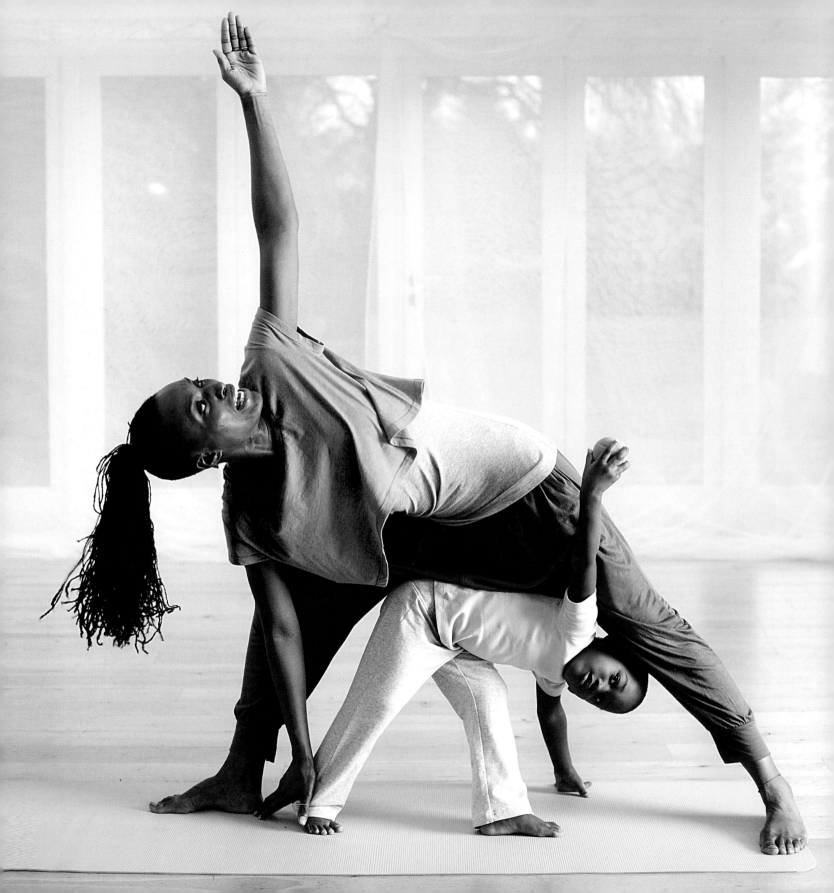

About this book

In our modern world, we learn the body language of baby care when we become parents. At the same time, new mothers face tremendous changes in their bodies and their lives. Within the vast array of yoga techniques for harmonizing body, mind, and spirit, this book presents an original set of simple practices to help mothers and babies find their very own way of being active together from birth to the third year. No previous experience of yoga is required. In joint playfulness with their mothers, yoga gives babies and toddlers an enjoyment of body movement that not only brings health benefits but also creates a sound foundation for self-confidence.

Birthlight is about the joy of being that is the ultimate goal of yoga, with a remit to promote this joy around pregnancy, birth, and babies from conception to early childhood. Whether in their blissful sleep or when they cry loud in distress, babies are our best yoga teachers. They inspire us to be calm, balanced, and centered. Baby yoga, as pioneered by Birthlight,

is an inclusive set of gentle body strokes, adapted yoga postures, moves for enhancing development, and playful interactive practices to enrich communication. Many combinations are possible to suit the needs of each mother and baby or toddler pair. Celebrating difference, honoring and accepting our babies' individual rhythms and needs, are central tenets of Birthlight, irrespective of parenting choices.

Like yoga, baby yoga is accessible to all. Its practice, gently and progressively, leads to a healthier lifestyle. Yoga adds ease, comfort, creativity, and fun to daily parent-baby interactions. The sight of a happy baby fills us with wonder. All babies in the world need both good food and loving touch. Baby massage and yoga help us to nurture our babies and in turn this nurtures and sometimes heals ourselves. Birthlight baby yoga comes with a debt of gratitude to the people who have taught me their traditional forms of closeness with babies around the world, most particularly grandmothers from India and the Amazon rainforest.

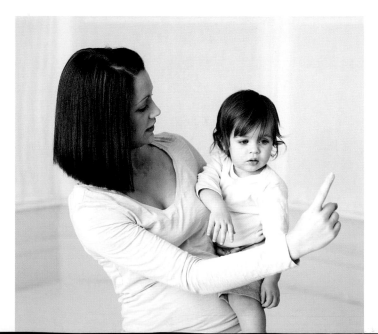

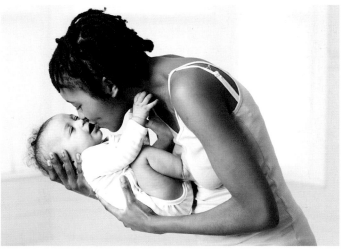

Where to start?

Your baby's mobility helps you to choose a starting point. If your baby is not yet mobile, it is best to follow the progressive practices from the beginning. Otherwise, starting from Chapter 5 will consolidate her skills, but she might also enjoy the soothing massage strokes and relaxing practices shown for younger babies.

In the west, baby massage and baby yoga adapted from India have developed into specific disciplines taught separately. This book follows the traditional Indian practice of combining them holistically from birth through their early years. If you feel unsure about starting with massage, relaxed holds and gentle moves may first help you get close to your new baby.

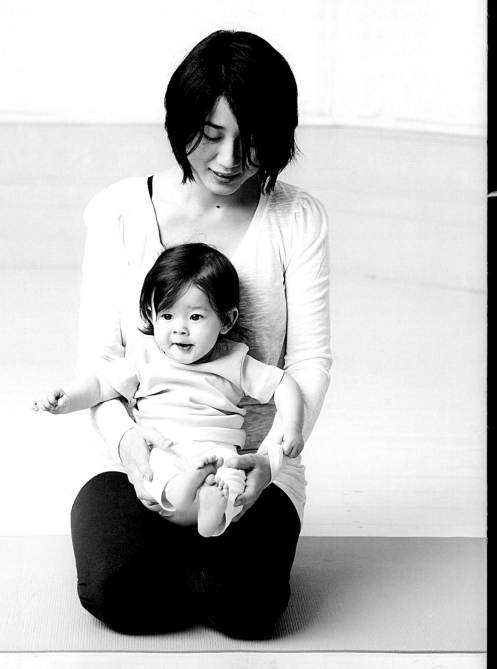

What your baby can do comfortably is more relevant than age for the choice of appropriate yoga moves. Unless you begin with your newborn, observe your baby's current abilities. Before trying massage strokes or yoga moves that appeal to you, practice making happy contact to develop positive associations. Each chapter includes similar sets of movements that are gradually more dynamic for older babies and toddlers—hip sequences, "tummy-time" stretches, mobility enhancers, rolls, balances, lifts, inversions, and relaxing practices. Resist offering your baby too much too soon. Watch his readiness to welcome and introduce new practices slowly, one by one.

The postnatal chapter includes your baby in your personal yoga practice. From early on in his life, your baby learns from watching and copying you. Your yoga, however basic, is an endless source of fun and inspiration for him and is also a way of establishing a healthy balance between your activities and your baby's demands. Babies come to accept, understand, and respect their mothers' practice as a special time for them, too.

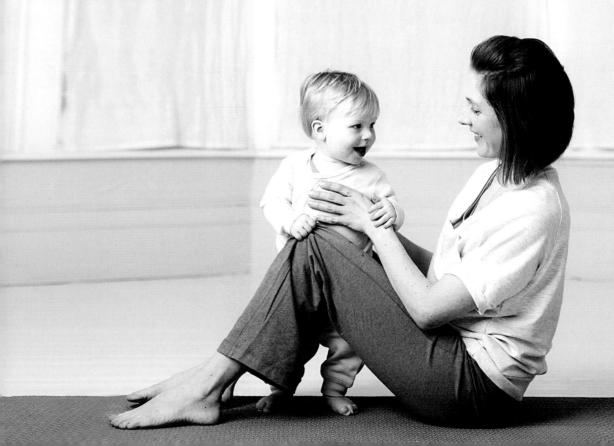

About the mothers

All the mothers in this book are featured with their own babies. Some had attended baby massage and yoga classes, others learnt practices on the spot. Most mothers had started yoga in pregnancy and were interested to continue, yet unsure about combining postnatal exercise with baby massage and baby yoga. Wherever you stand along the continuum, from mothers completely new to yoga to the four experienced yoga practitioners and teachers who modeled for this book, it is reassuring that the practices featured suited all the mother-baby pairs, irrespective of fitness or skills.

Just like on any day with babies and toddlers at home, our photo shoot followed alternating times of activity and rest, excitement and frustration, strife and breakthroughs. It was truly wonderful to see that there were massage and yoga practices to suit all moods. As they left, mothers smiled more than when they first arrived. Even short sequences offered them new opportunities to interact with their babies.

Most of all perhaps, babies and toddlers relished a free space to perform their latest skills. Simple baby yoga moves proved invaluable in offering effective support to premobile babies. One baby rolled over for the first time. Another took off in spectacular crawling a few minutes after his mother said he had been static on all-fours for weeks. Everyone present rejoiced.

Are we understimulating babies, or overwhelming them with visual and auditory stimuli that limit the potential body-based communication we could have with them? A bare yoga mat offers a blank space where babies can show us how they grow and learn, and also guide us to best help them.

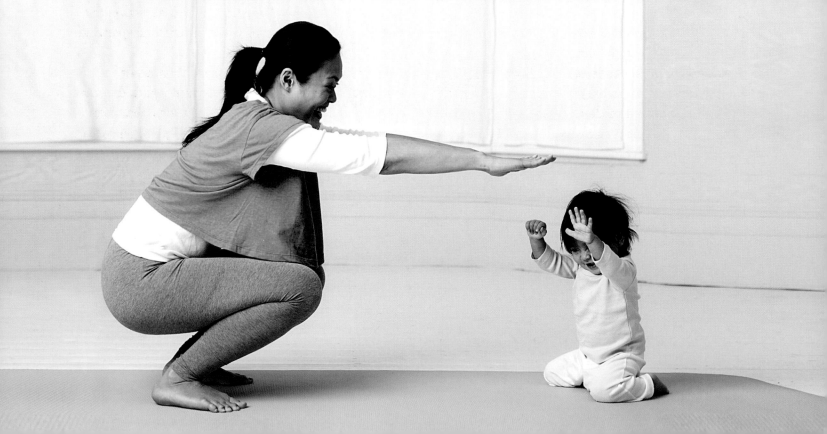

Why do baby massage and yoga?

Massage and yoga are practical ways of communicating love and affection to babies, when scientific research is progressively revealing how much babies need touch and movement for the healthy development of their brains. The sense of touch develops in the fourth week in the womb, but it takes two years from birth to establish the brain connections that enable rational and caring responses. This wiring is largely based on life experiences. Touch brings with it connection and communication, stimulation and relaxation, calming and healing. Babies need quality interaction with the adults closest to them to feel secure and free to explore.

In urban industrialized environments, babies are most often separated from their parents' bodies and kept still in cribs, carriers, and seats. Baby yoga moves are, first of all, a way to recreate active closeness, a structured mode of relating dynamically with babies, very gently at first and then within the greater range of movement they seek. Enhancing the vestibular system, the part of our brain that coordinates our spatial awareness, sets a foundation for good posture, balance, flexibility, and agility.

Physical effects

Digestion, a most important and delicate process for newborns, is best eased and regulated by touch and gentle movement combined. While there is no ready treatment for colic, relaxed holds and walking can help parents to calm their distressed babies (and also themselves) effectively. Gas and constipation are common complaints that respond readily to massage and yoga, to the great relief of affected babies. The wide array of soothing and entertaining moves also eases the dilemma many new mothers experience between resorting to frequent feeding or letting babies cry between routine feeds.

Easier digestion and appropriate physical stimulation contribute to better sleep, which in turns promotes growth and contentment, bringing out your baby's irresistible charm. Massage is known to deepen and regulate breathing as well as improving blood circulation, both of which promote deeper and longer sleep.

If crying, sleep deprivation, and hopeless exhaustion have settled in, and cause you to despair when you pick up this book, do not lose heart. An abundance of easy practices can help you reverse this spiral of doom and gloom into an expanding positive spiral of joy and wellbeing. The effects of a more comfortable hold, a foot massage, or simple hip movements on your baby's physiology can lift her mood. As she smiles, your cheering response will reassure her that all is well, which in turn will increase her inner security.

Physiological benefits

During pregnancy and around birth, new mothers experience a release of the hormone oxytocin, associated with relaxation, connection, and nurturing. Baby massage and yoga both stimulate the ongoing positive effects of this hormone, and loving touch also helps you to regulate stress hormones, such as cortisol. Love at first sight between mothers and newborns is actually unusual, particularly after challenging births, and this magic bonding is something best brought about day by day. The more often you massage and do yoga with your baby, the greater the combined sensory effects that enhance closeness.

Yoga is about developing self-awareness. Registering how stress affects us and can be communicated to babies unwittingly is the foundation of joint parent-baby relaxation. Once you notice how your baby is more likely to fuss while you are preparing dinner or are about to go out, you can use instant relaxation practices to reassure her and slow down. Applied to the many small separations and reunions that are experienced as your baby grows, positive touch and yoga can reinforce a secure sense of stable continuity.

While mothers are often advised not to massage their babies when they are affected by negative emotions, such as anger or anxiety, the Birthlight approach encourages you to trust the power of positive transformation together with your baby. Through easy practices, such as walking relaxation, rhythmical gentle rocking, and massage, with rhymes that open the throat and lighten the heart, it is possible to engage physically with your baby and reconnect with the love and wonder right there in front of you. Of course, it may not be so simple, but it is worth trying. As your confidence in handling your baby develops, you are more likely to perceive yourself as a wonderful mum whom your baby simply adores even when she is cranky. Exercising together with your baby will also give you more energy.

Can you put yourself in your baby's booties? Massage and yoga raise your awareness of your baby's overall enjoyment of quieter or more energetic activities. With regular practice, you are creating a framework in which your baby can better regulate her own levels of physical and emotional arousal, attention and concentration, interest in the world or withdrawal.

As babies grow into toddlers, the yoga mat can be a neutral space where emotions can be expressed safely, boundaries negotiated, and lasting trust built through a more complex interaction involving touch, movement, language, and imagination.

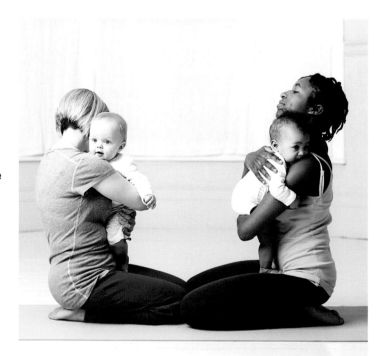

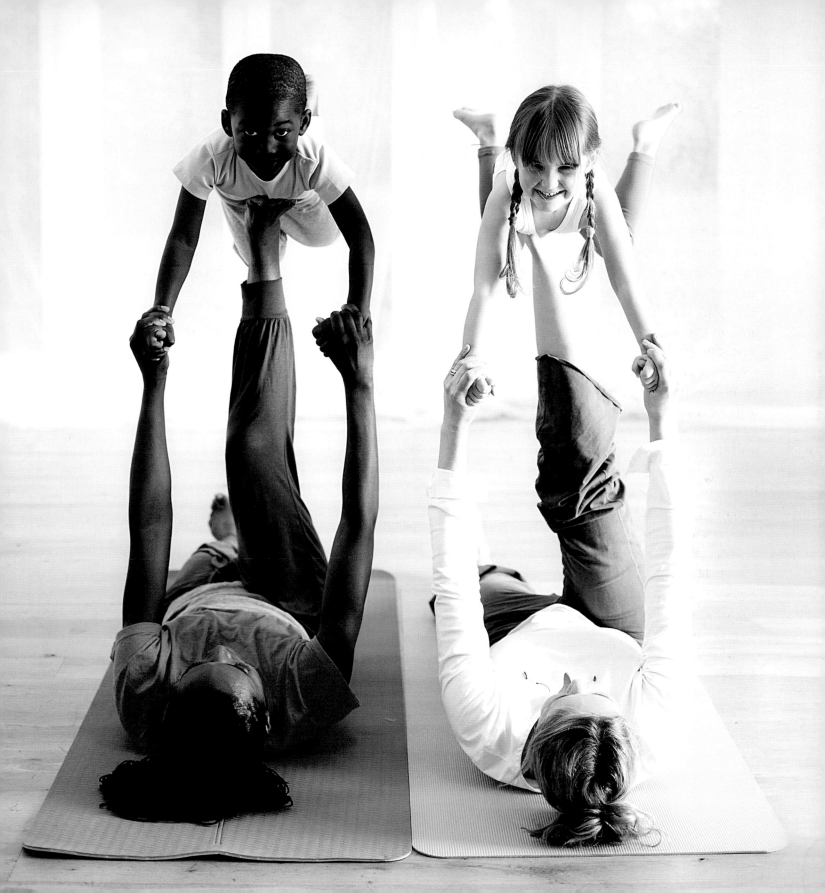

Where and when to do baby massage and yoga

A classic mat creates the yoga space through this book, but rural Indian mothers do not have mats. No equipment is indispensible. After ensuring your baby's willingness and comfort—temperature matters most—you are ready to start. If your baby objects to a particular step in a sequence, avoid it for a few days and then introduce it again within the sequence. Acceptance and patience are the qualities you most need to cultivate in order to face the unpredictability of early practices and inevitable frequent interruptions. What your baby will remember most is how cherished and valued she felt during this quality time with you.

Interpreting your baby's cues

First check your baby's receptivity to touch and movement before engaging with her. Responding to her "Yes" or "No" cues is paramount.

- Babies say YES to massage and yoga when they are open and responsive in an awake, alert state, shown by gazing with open eyes, reaching out, cooing, smiling, and moving their legs and arms harmoniously. It is ideal to start massaging a baby in this state.

- Babies say NO to massage or yoga with their bodies—they turn away, cry, yawn, or hiccup, wrinkle their foreheads, and grimace with their faces. If not listened to, they may produce stronger signals, such as kicking and pulling away, arching their backs, turning paler or redder, and of course crying louder. They can also extend one arm in front of their face as if to say STOP, splay out their hands and feet away from their bodies in a bracing action, or show sudden alternate flexing and tensing of arms and legs. Shifts from placid to erratic states also express refusal. Less visibly, babies may withdraw and show no response whatsoever, an extreme form of disengagement that needs to be acknowledged.

How long?

On days when you have time and your baby is receptive, there may be an opportunity for a long practice. Otherwise, a short practice can be fun-packed, and instant practices of 1–3 minutes will enhance your interaction with your baby or toddler at any time.

- Short practice, 5–10 minutes: This is ideal for babies under four months, at home before bath time but also possibly away from home during the day. A mat or special cloth or fleece can mark the setting. You can signal beginnings and endings with markers of your choice, such as a song or a gesture.

- Long practice, 10–30 minutes: This is preferably done at home, and is a perfect time for integrating massage, yoga moves, and relaxation for babies over four months. A dedicated setting and clear markers help regular practice.

If your baby is not very enthusiastic but does not manifest any of the listed NO cues, start tentatively and be prepared to stop. Babies are clear but vulnerable; it is our responsibility as adults to learn to decipher their signals.

Are you ready?

Go through a basic self-checklist. Are you comfortable? Are you showing attunement with your baby with eye contact, facial expression, and a softer and slower voice? Telling your baby what you are doing, setting the space for joint practice, or centering yourself with three breaths can be ways of showing her that you are ready to make yourself fully available to her. Many babies have a great sense of humor and welcome small surprises and jokes, once a relaxed and steady routine has been established. If your joint practice has been interrupted for more than a few days for any reason, always go back to the activities that your baby enjoyed before you stopped.

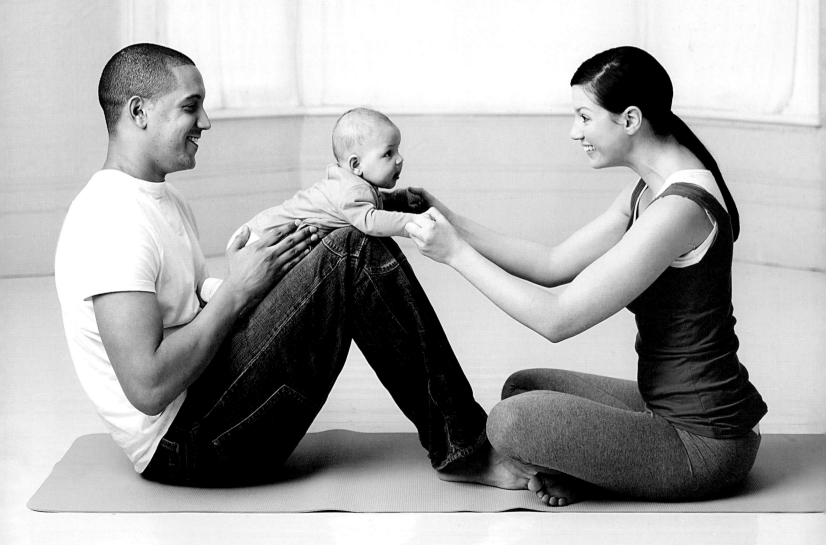

Getting ready

Have you noticed that when you feel calm, your baby also tends to be calm? Music can help you achieve that composure. Choose something you find relaxing and, ideally, sing along. It is the rhythmical aspect of both music and speech that babies engage with—voices softer, slower, and a higher pitch than normal. Babies respond to tonal variations and emotions in your voice from soon after birth, and are able to follow rhythms long before they learn to speak. They soon associate words and actions through repetitions, so tell your baby what you are going to do, or sing a simple rhyme. Your baby will take part in the "conversation" in ways that will become gradually more perceptible to you. Don't be in a rush, though, because babies' ability to deal with outside stimuli develops progressively in order to avoid sensory overload.

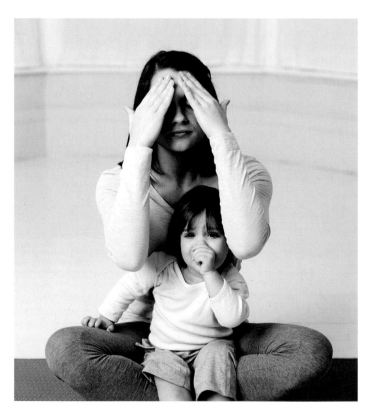

1 Start with massaging your forehead, using your three middle fingers on both hands.

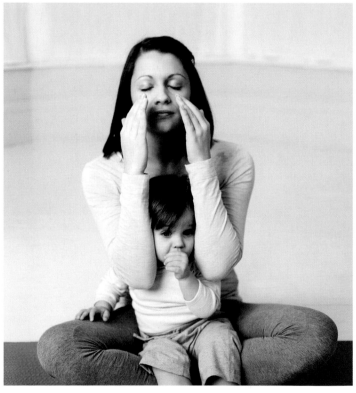

2 Trace a line from the side of your nose, about halfway down, above your cheekbones.

Create a relaxed environment

Before you start, it's important to make the space to focus on your baby whatever happens outside. Get rid of tension or anxiety by stamping your feet for a few seconds, and shaking your hands. Make fists and open them saying "Ha" as you do so. Ask yourself if you are emotionally available, that is ready to be absorbed in the activity with your baby, and in tune with it and him. Are you relaxed enough to synchronize with your baby, and calm enough to regulate his emotional states? Ask, "Am I ready to watch, listen, observe, and learn from my baby?"

It is important that you feel comfortable, so if you do not feel right sitting on the floor, prepare to massage your baby while sitting at a table, or use a couch or a low bed.

Your natural scent is your baby's favorite, so don't wear perfume. Take off your shoes and center yourself by taking three deep breaths. Close and open your eyes three times, relax your lower jaw, and rotate your shoulders a few times forward and backward. Place your hands on your heart and feel connection to all you love.

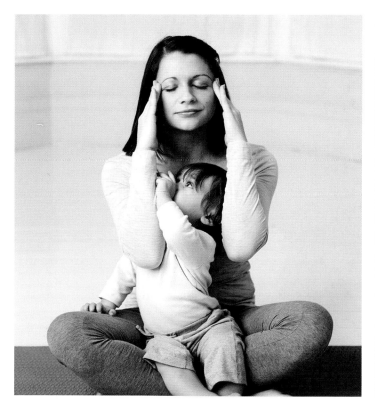

3 Continue with small circular movements of your fingers on your temples, round the dip that you find above the top of your jaw bone. Inward circles are most relaxing.

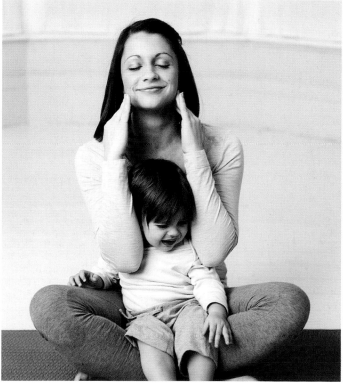

4 Glide your hands down to your lower jaw. With a gentle stroke be aware of your glands and relax any tension in your lower jaw. This often releases a smile, too.

Basic holds

After the dramatic transition from the confinement of the womb to a boundless world, most babies find it comforting to be held in a firm yet relaxed position, head and back supported, that reproduces the fetal containment of their limbs. Cradling is the first and most basic way of making your baby feel secure and content in your arms. Relaxed holds have the same effect, and also help babies to uncurl their spines. Whether or not you have already fallen in love with your baby by this stage, early and prolonged close contact helps to develop a lasting bond. You will soon recognize when your baby is in an alert albeit fussy frame of mind, or in need of sleep rather than being aroused to a more responsive state. Enjoy practicing these holds until you feel comfortable shifting from one to another with as few movements as possible.

Just stroking your baby gently while supporting her in a basic hold can be very calming.

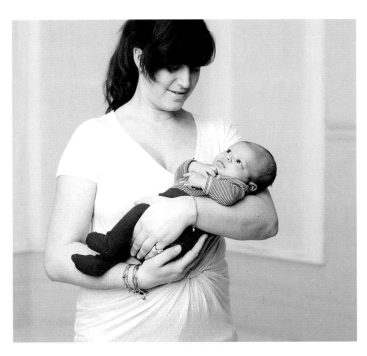

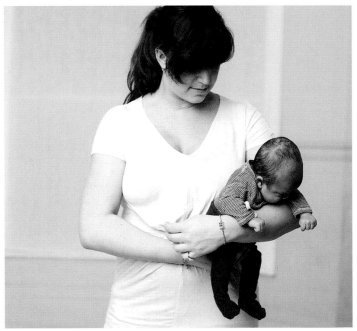

Cradle hold

With elbows softly bent, hold your baby against you in the crook of one arm, hand around her thigh, while supporting her bottom and back with the other hand. The cradle hold and cradle rocking—continuous gentle movement of your body from side to side—are a source of pleasure for babies.

Safety hold

Use one arm as a banister for your baby to lean on, and the other hand—the "seat" hand—to support her bottom. As she grows, you can extend your banister arm, holding the baby with your thumb and index finger under her armpit in a secure cleft grip. This will give you more freedom of movement.

Shoulder hold

For this soothing hold—often a favorite with fathers—make sure that your baby's chest rests on your chest or shoulder so as to ensure natural head balance. For a very young baby, you may wish to hold her head as additional support.

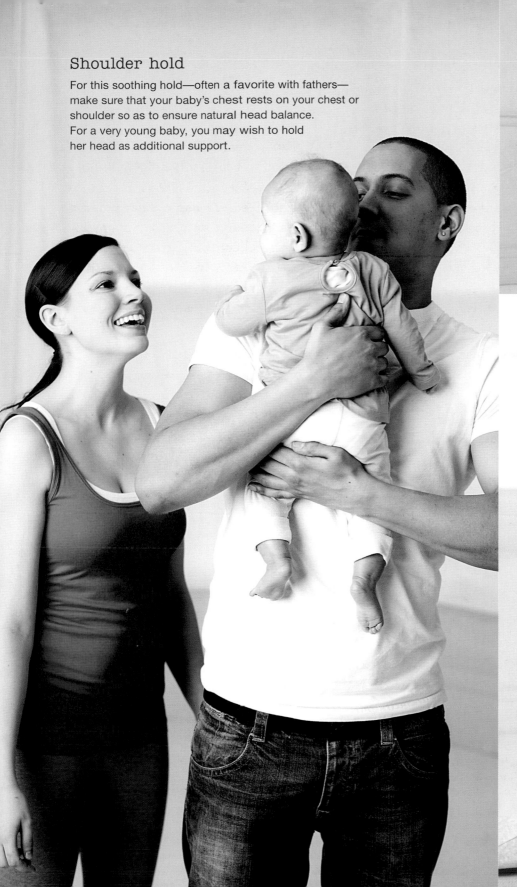

One-arm relaxed hold

Once you are confident with these three holds, and secure with aligning your baby's body, you can hold her safely using just one arm. Sit her on your hip by holding her between her legs with your arm over her shoulder. To return to a cradle hold, slide her into a horizontal position across your body and support her bottom and back with your other hand.

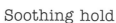

Soothing hold

From a cradle hold, roll your baby's body carefully so that his back is toward you, and extend your hand between his legs so that you can stroke his stomach very gently. Your other hand should envelop his shoulder and arm. This is an ideal hold for babies who experience pain after feeding, or tend to have hiccups or reflux. Walking slowly and rhythmically while holding your baby like this is a good way to induce sleep.

Self-winding hold

Many people around the world let their babies wind themselves by supporting them in a vertical position. Try sitting your baby, even newborn, on your thigh, supporting her with your hands, back and front. Spread your front hand across her upper chest and hold her face from ear to ear between your thumb and index finger. You can then rub her back gently upward if she does not wind herself.

Contained holds

Most babies can benefit from feeling "contained" when they are very tired or upset, and while swaddling, as still practiced in some parts of the world, remains controversial, contained holds are not. These enveloping holds are particularly helpful in calming sensitive babies who can easily become agitated and whose crying rapidly escalates. In addition, while helping your baby to feel safe and secure, you also become calmer and are more likely to feel that you are meeting your baby's needs.

Contained head cradle

After any intervention that has caused your baby pain, or when he ends a bout of crying, or for extra comfort at any time, try this hold. Sitting cross-legged, lay him securely across your lap and, with your arm lightly resting down the side of his body, gently hold his shoulder while cupping his head with your other hand. When he is calm, move into the instant relaxation hold.

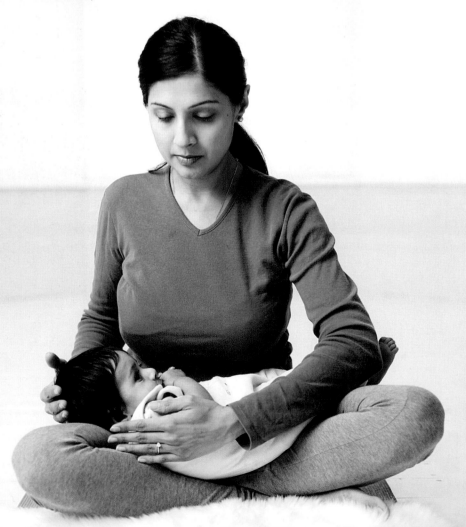

Rocking the cradle

Sit cross-legged and cocoon your baby securely in your arms, holding his feet together. Rock him gently up and down, talking softly to him all the while to reassure him that all is well.

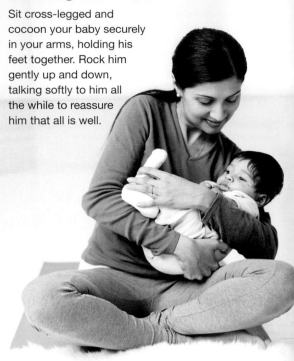

Instant relaxation hold

With your baby on your lap, gently rest your chin on his head while holding his feet firmly for a couple of minutes. Release and repeat two or three times until you feel him relaxing. You could rest one hand on your baby's head and hold his feet with the other hand, if you prefer, and you could also do this while he is lying on his back.

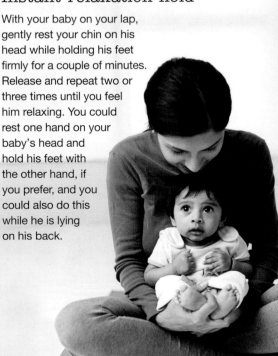

1 Baby Massage

Once you feel confident holding your baby, you can start to introduce massage into her routine slowly. Progress from initial hand contact to stroking while she is fully dressed, gradually moving on to body massage with oil. If your baby dislikes being undressed, start with foot massage, or try the dry strokes that open the first hip sequence (page 37). In any case, massage her feet and legs first to build trust before going on to massage the body. From about six weeks old, most babies enjoy a full massage, introduced over a period of about two weeks.

Baby massage is based on two simple techniques. Long strokes using the palms of your hands in slow, firm, and continuous movements—effleurage—come first. Even the youngest babies enjoy a firm touch. As a rule, apply relatively stronger pressure as you move toward the heart, lighter on the return. Take your time to find an easy rhythm, and try to keep one of your hands in contact with your baby's body at all times.

The second technique consists of small circular movements—frictions—using the pads of your thumbs and fingers over small areas, particularly on feet, hands, and face. Start with light movements, making them progressively deeper to your baby's liking.

Together you and your baby are discovering how she likes being massaged. Keep watching for cues (page 14) to see when, and where, she is responsive or resistant to your touch. Adjust your massage to her moods and preferences. Brisker strokes will improve muscle tone while slower, gentler strokes are calming and relaxing.

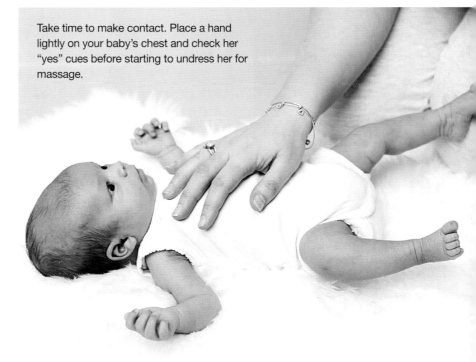

Take time to make contact. Place a hand lightly on your baby's chest and check her "yes" cues before starting to undress her for massage.

Lower body massage

Most babies prefer body massage to start with long strokes down and up their legs, followed by small strokes on their feet and around their abdomen.

Relax and engage your mind fully in your loving touch, suspend any lack of self-confidence, and trust that you can do this well.

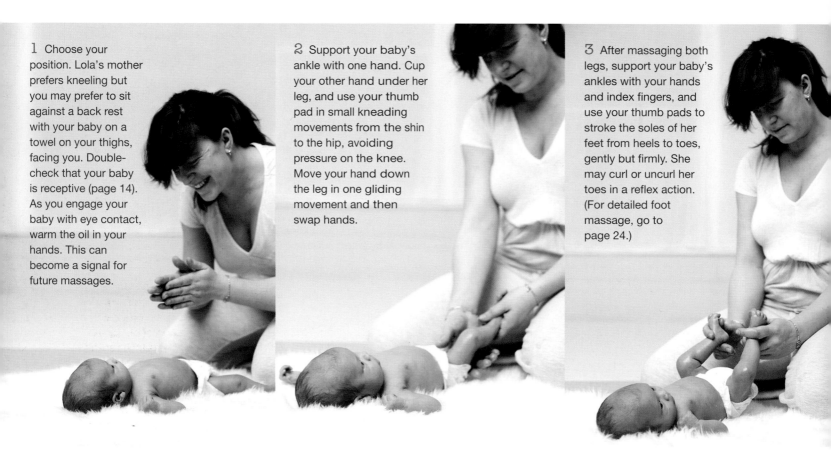

1 Choose your position. Lola's mother prefers kneeling but you may prefer to sit against a back rest with your baby on a towel on your thighs, facing you. Double-check that your baby is receptive (page 14). As you engage your baby with eye contact, warm the oil in your hands. This can become a signal for future massages.

2 Support your baby's ankle with one hand. Cup your other hand under her leg, and use your thumb pad in small kneading movements from the shin to the hip, avoiding pressure on the knee. Move your hand down the leg in one gliding movement and then swap hands.

3 After massaging both legs, support your baby's ankles with your hands and index fingers, and use your thumb pads to stroke the soles of her feet from heels to toes, gently but firmly. She may curl or uncurl her toes in a reflex action. (For detailed foot massage, go to page 24.)

Using oil

To reduce irritation and make strokes more comfortable, use an organic or cold-pressed vegetable oil—sunflower oil or fractionated coconut oil are good for baby massage, and are easy to obtain and store. Don't use mineral oils, because they are petroleum based, or essential oils, even lavender, due to their possible effects on babies' nervous and immune systems. Also, don't use a prescribed emollient cream for massage, particularly toward the heart and against hair growth.

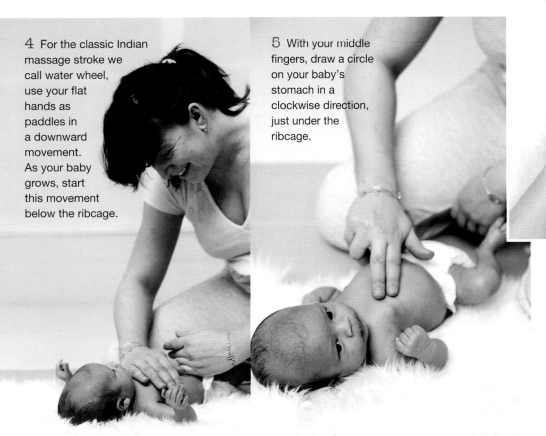

4 For the classic Indian massage stroke we call water wheel, use your flat hands as paddles in a downward movement. As your baby grows, start this movement below the ribcage.

5 With your middle fingers, draw a circle on your baby's stomach in a clockwise direction, just under the ribcage.

6 Without lifting your baby's bottom, slide your hands under her lower back from the sides. Using both hands, stroke down the back of the legs to the ankles and finish with a gentle ankle hold. This is enough for a first massage. You may want to practice this sequence for a few days so that it becomes a relaxed routine for you and your baby.

Precautions

- Do not massage your baby while he is asleep or just after a feed. Wait at least 30 minutes after feeding because the activity draws blood to the skin and away from the digestive organs.
- Avoid massage if your baby has a fever, has injuries resulting in bruising and swelling, has open wounds or rashes, has undergone recent surgery, and for three days after vaccination.
- Start massaging newborns only when their navels have healed and there are no signs of jaundice. Be careful of overstimulation Build up to a full ten-minute routine gradually, and make sure he can cope with, and is enjoying, each stage as you go along.
- If your baby's hips click or seem unstable, it is advisable to have them checked by your doctor.

Foot massage

The practice of reflexology is based on the theory that parts of the body can be stimulated through concentrating on specific points on the feet. So massaging the whole of your baby's foot may induce beneficial effects for the rest of the body, enhancing digestion, relaxing the solar plexus, easing teething pains, and helping with nasal and ear congestion. Gently massage each foot in turn.

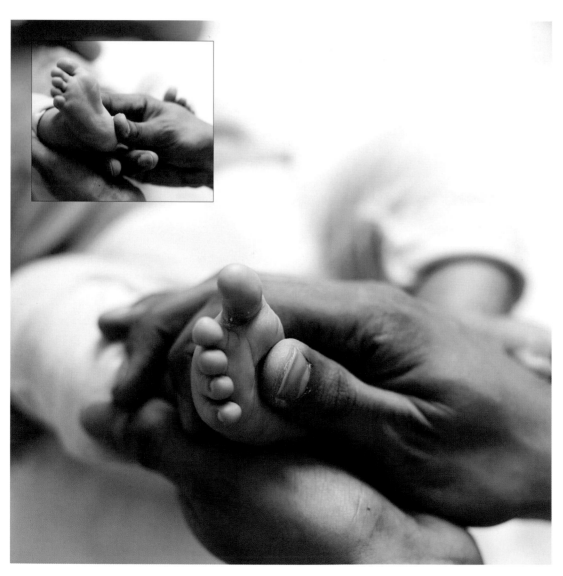

1 Support the ankle with one hand, and move the thumb of your other hand up the sole of your baby's foot, using small outward strokes. There is a soft spot at the center of your baby's foot, which in eastern traditions is known as the "bubbling spring." Press it gently for a few seconds before continuing your upward stroke.

Glide your hand back to the heel and repeat three times.

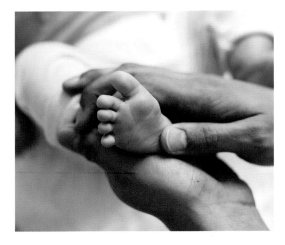

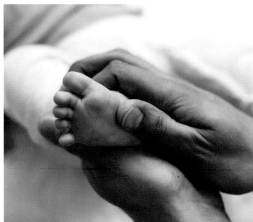

2 Follow the dip above your baby's heel with your thumb pad from the outside to the inside arch. Repeat three times. This is beneficial for your baby's digestion.

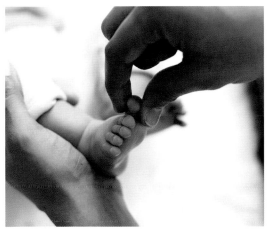

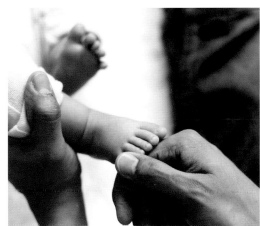

3 Starting with the big toe, roll your index finger and thumb from base to tip. Press your fingers gently when you reach the toe's tip. Repeat on all the toes.

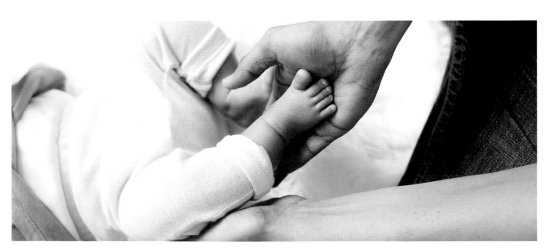

4 After you have completed all the strokes, gently hold your baby's leg while resting her foot in the palm of your hand for a few seconds. Breathe deeply and relax.

Upper body massage

Reaching your baby's heart through touch triggers a cascade of happy chemicals in her brain as she feels nurtured and loved. Adjust pressure carefully, starting with a very light touch at first. Respect your baby's resistance at any time, and remember to smile at her, especially if she seems tentative.

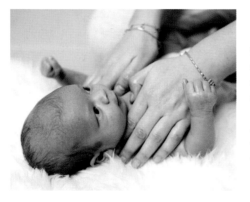

1 Place both your hands flat on your baby's chest. Again, check that your baby is receptive. Some babies take longer to welcome chest massage.

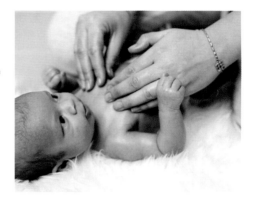

2 Using both hands, try small strokes up the middle of your baby's chest toward her neck. If your baby is happy, continue. If she responds with tension, move to Step 4.

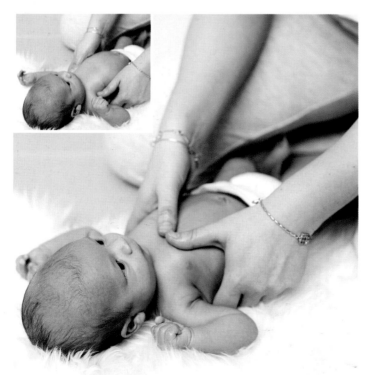

3 With your thumb pads, trace small semicircles up toward your baby's neck, down to the sides, and then back to the center.

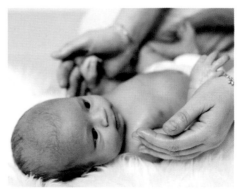

4 Slide your hands onto your baby's shoulders. With a long smooth stroke, glide your hands to her hands. If your baby is relaxed she may open her palms, but never force her to do so.

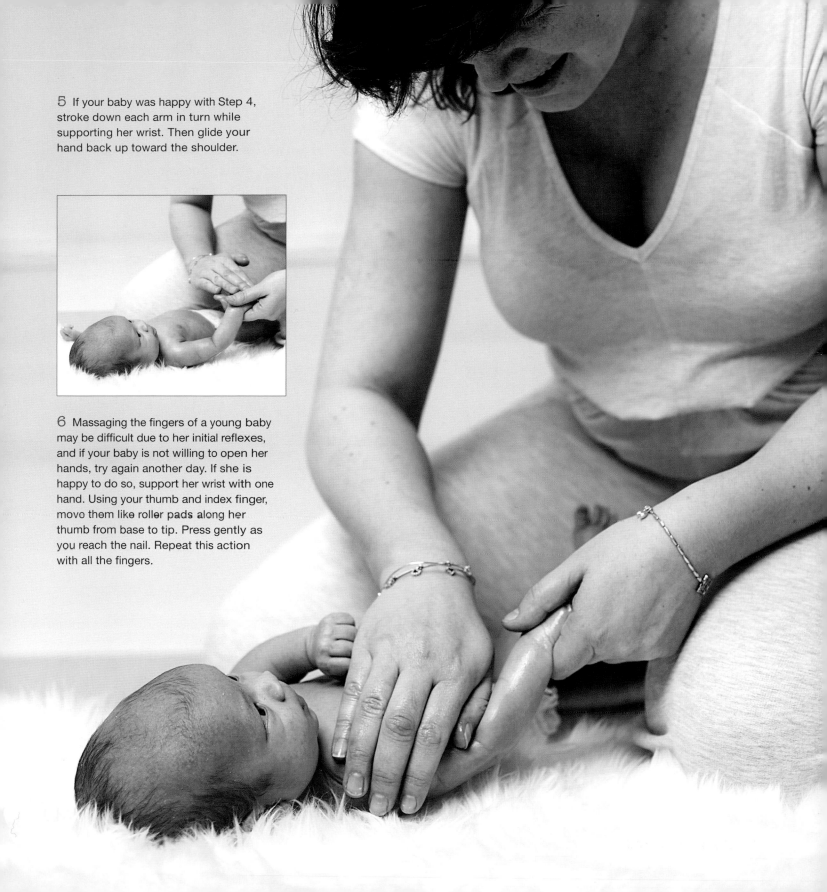

5 If your baby was happy with Step 4, stroke down each arm in turn while supporting her wrist. Then glide your hand back up toward the shoulder.

6 Massaging the fingers of a young baby may be difficult due to her initial reflexes, and if your baby is not willing to open her hands, try again another day. If she is happy to do so, support her wrist with one hand. Using your thumb and index finger, move them like roller pads along her thumb from base to tip. Press gently as you reach the nail. Repeat this action with all the fingers.

Head and face massage

Your baby's face is extremely sensitive. Each gentle movement of your fingers on her forehead, repeated several times, induces relaxation responses leading to blissful sleep.

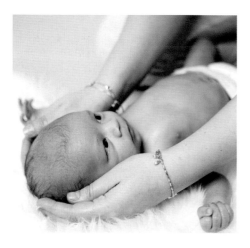

1 Cup your baby's head with both hands. Check that she is happy.

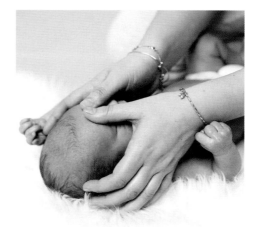

2 With your thumb pads make small circular movements from her forehead, extending to the sides of her head, ending behind the ears. Repeat three times.

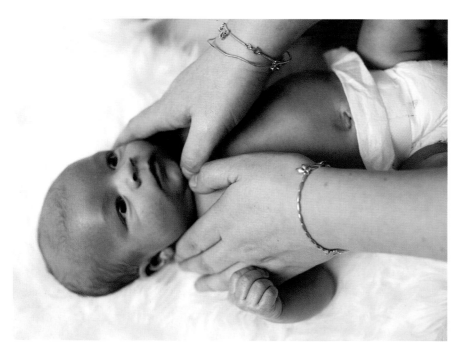

3 Stroke her chin with your thumb pads. If she is happy, stroke outward from the sides of the nose toward her ears along the base of the cheekbones. Be careful—a touch on the cheeks may prompt your baby to open her mouth and expect a feed.

Back stroke

Newborns may not be ready for a back massage until their spines have uncurled in the second month.

Always make sure that a young baby's airway is clear with her head to one side or another.

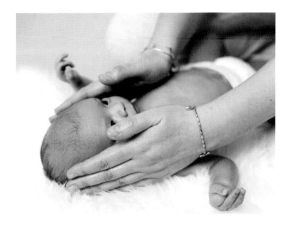

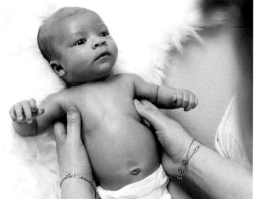

End your newborn's massage with a long back stroke, gliding your flat hands from the sides of her head, under her shoulders and arms, all the way down to her buttocks and legs. Repeat three times. Slow and calming strokes signal the end of massage to your baby and may induce sleep.

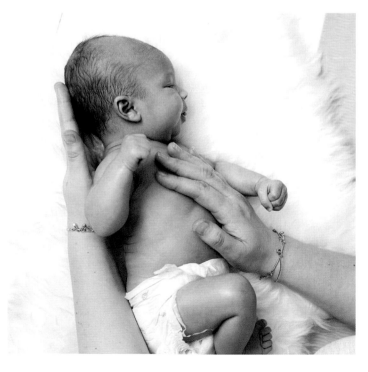

Alternately, with your baby on her side, you may glide one hand down from the top of her head to her lower back while pressing gently on her chest with the flat of your other hand. This has a containing effect that may encourage your baby to feel secure, and help her fall asleep.

Singing

This is an ideal time to start singing to your baby. Choose your favorite nursery rhyme or invent a new song for her. For months, and even a couple of years to come, you will be her diva, however out of tune you are when you sing to her. She will love even the most basic rhymes, which have been shown to boost brain development irrespective of the singer's skills.

Massage for wind, colic, & constipation

Colic is still mysterious. Not considered a medical condition, it is nevertheless distressing to both babies and helpless parents—reflux, or regurgitating food, is even more so. These ailments will eventually disappear and, in the meantime, massage can help make your baby more comfortable. It is not just a question of technique. Your anxiety is inevitably communicated to your baby, so if you can relax—and massaging your baby will help ease your own tension—you will be able to help him more effectively.

Caution

- Check with your doctor or health visitor that your baby's abdominal pain is due to wind, colic, or constipation, or whether there may be any other possible reason for it.
- Do not massage your baby during bouts of colic. The best time is half an hour to an hour before the usual onset of colicky crying (probably late afternoon), before your baby is in pain.

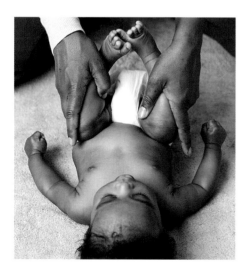

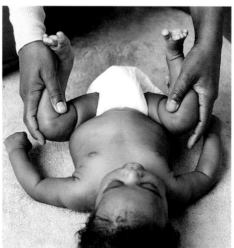

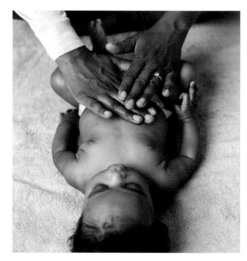

1 Before starting massage, place your hands on his shins and gently press his legs toward his body, then release, three times. This "knees to tummy" action may alleviate tension or pain.

2 If your baby is happy, continue with circular outward movements of his legs, also three times. Be careful not to lift your baby's bottom off the mat throughout.

3 Now place your hands on your baby's tummy, one on top of the other, and feel whether it is hard or bloated. Adjust the pressure depending on your baby's response, making it lighter if he frowns. With the flat of one hand, and keeping the other hand on top to maintain the pressure, stroke under the line of your baby's ribcage clockwise three times.

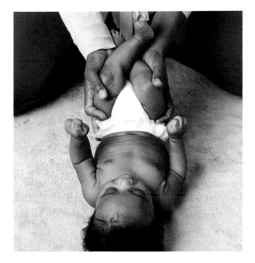

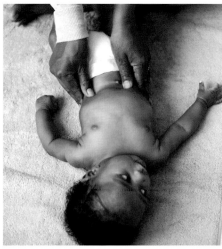

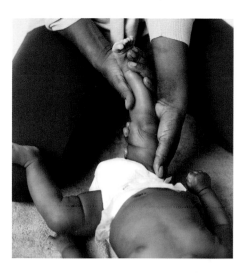

4 Glide your hands to the sides of your baby's hips and support the back of his thighs. With gentle but firm pressure, cross his legs alternately, taking care not to lift his buttocks off the mat.

5 With your hands holding your baby's lower back and sides, use your thumb pads to stroke outward from the middle of his tummy below the navel. Repeat three times to alleviate constipation.

6 Massaging the leg will also help. Hold your baby's ankle with one hand and his thigh with the other, allowing the thumb to extend high up toward the hip (avoid pressing near the groin). Glide your hand back to your baby's ankle, using the thumb quite firmly.

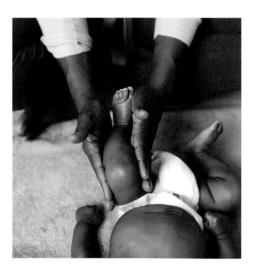

8 To end the massage, alternately bend and extend your baby's legs—like a piston. Hold his legs firmly under the knees and find a rhythm that suits his age and disposition. Most babies enjoy stronger movements than we offer them. Traditional baby massage is surprisingly energetic.

At the end of this practice, wrap up your baby to keep him warm and take a moment for relaxation. If he gets fussy, walk with him in a soothing hold (page 19.) Repeat this sequence each day for best results

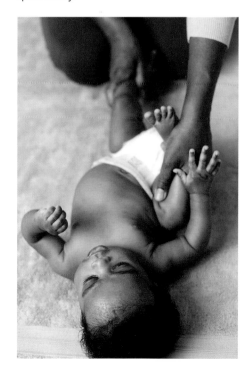

7 Add a rolling stroke to relax the whole of your baby's leg. Take his leg between your palms and move your hands up and down, as if you were making a pastry roll. Go gently over the knee and ankle joints as you repeat the "rolly."

Opening the chest

This sequence combines front and back massage to help ease congestion in your baby's chest. It is very helpful as a preventive if there is a history of asthma in the family. Using oil facilitates this sequence. Stroke his back gently in shoulder hold (page 19) through the day.

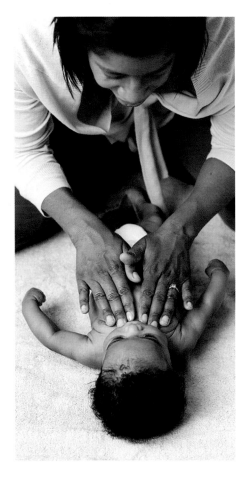 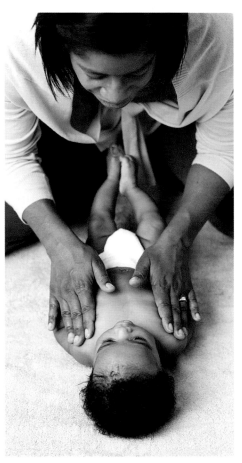 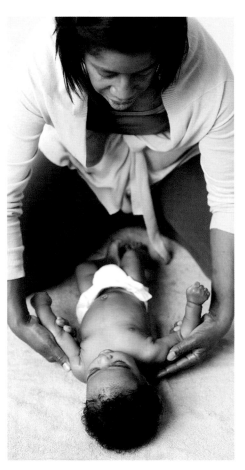

1 Place both your hands flat on your baby's chest and rub gently up and down with your finger pads.

2 With your thumbs on your baby's sternum at the center of his chest, spread the flat of your hands to the sides with a gentle and even pressure. Release the pressure as you glide your hands back to center. Repeat three times.

3 Cup your hands under your baby's shoulders and gently stroke down his arms to the wrists with a relaxed slow movement so that he does not tense up. Repeat three times.

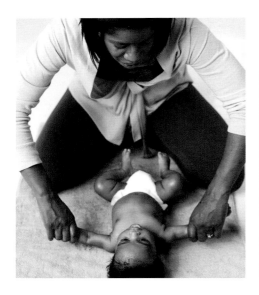

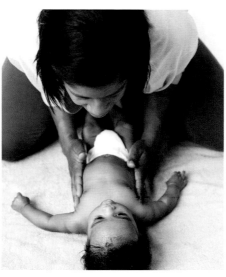

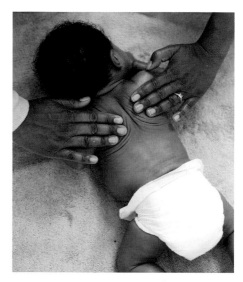

4 If your baby is happy, hold his upper arms with your fingers above and your thumbs below his arms. Slide your hands toward his wrists using small up and down movements. The aim is to open out his arms fully. Repeat three times.

5 From the center of his chest, glide your hands to the sides of his ribcage and reach around to the back ribs with your fingers. Your baby may enjoy small rolling movements as you use a slight pressure on alternate sides.

6 Turn your baby over onto his belly and make sure he is comfortable. Rub his upper back with your palms, up and down from his neck, pressing gently with your finger pads.

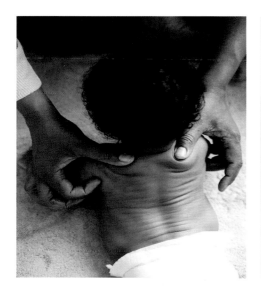

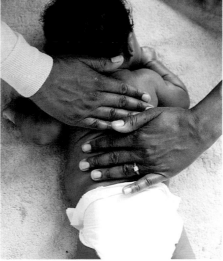

9 Rub plenty of oil into your hands. Place one hand on one of your baby's shoulders and your other hand on his waist on the opposite side. Using your finger pads, stroke away from the spine, applying gentle pressure, and glide back to the center, avoiding contact with the spine at all times. After your hands meet in the middle of your baby's back, keep massaging and repeat once.

At the end of this massage, wrap your baby warmly and give him a cuddle.

7 If he enjoys the pressure, make small circles with your thumb pads at the base of his neck from the center to the sides.

8 Use your hands as paddles to stroke from his shoulders down his back—away from you if he is facing you, toward you if he is facing away from you. Repeat a few times.

Positive touch

All of baby massage involves a positive use of touch.
Here are some additional practices that babies find
calming and securing.

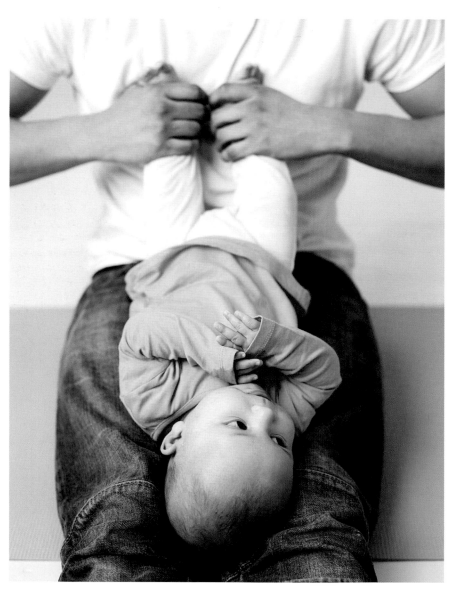

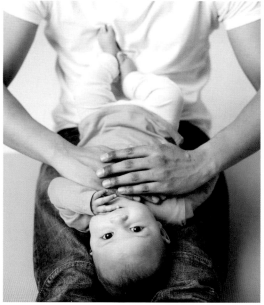

Feet hold

Holding a baby's feet firmly, one in each hand,
can be securing for babies who move their legs
and arms a lot when they cry, or try to calm
themselves by placing their hands over their
faces, or resist cuddles and avoid eye contact.
It is also an easy way of saying "I love you" if you
feel upset and not ready to engage with your
baby at this time. Finish by placing your hands
gently on her chest.

Calming points on your baby's face

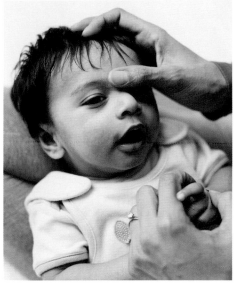 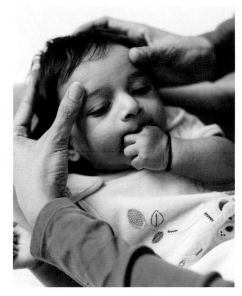 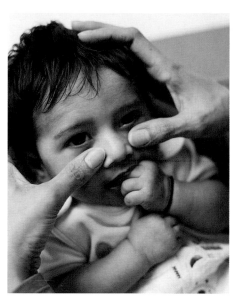

● Nose stroke. Gently press the point between your baby's eyebrows using your thumb pad, and stroke down his nose in a short repetitive movement. This practice is used to help babies fall asleep across many cultures.

● Forehead stroke. Cup your baby's head with both hands and position your thumbs flat at the center of his forehead. Slowly stroke his forehead from the center to the temples, gliding your thumbs back to the center. Repeat the stroke until he gradually closes his eyes, which will ease his transition into sleep.

● Nose wings. Gently press your thumb pads on each side of your baby's nostrils, and make a short stroke downward and sideways under the cheekbones. This is helpful when babies are fretful because of mucus collected in their noses, and is also generally conducive to better breathing.

Ear massage

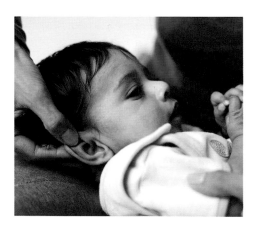

Using your thumb and index finger, press along the rim of your baby's ear, from the top of the ear to the lobe. Think of small stitches. Finish with small round movements on the lobe, applying gentle pressure. Auricular massage is an ancient eastern technique that is used to balance all the body systems and it can be used safely on babies.

2 First Moves

Touch and movement are complementary. Most people around the world start with baby massage, but ours is not a massage culture in which we routinely use touch to promote each other's wellbeing beyond simple hugs. If your baby did not respond well to your first massage attempts, or baby massage did not feel easy for you to initiate, baby yoga might be a better option for engaging with your baby in a physical, body-based communication from birth. One practice will inevitably facilitate the other, whichever you start with. Baby massage will help you and your baby to relax together and baby yoga will stimulate your baby to explore her range of movement in sheer enjoyment. Gradually, you will gain the confidence to combine massage and yoga in versatile and creative ways to suit your baby's particular needs at different times of day and at various stages of development, and to suit each other's moods.

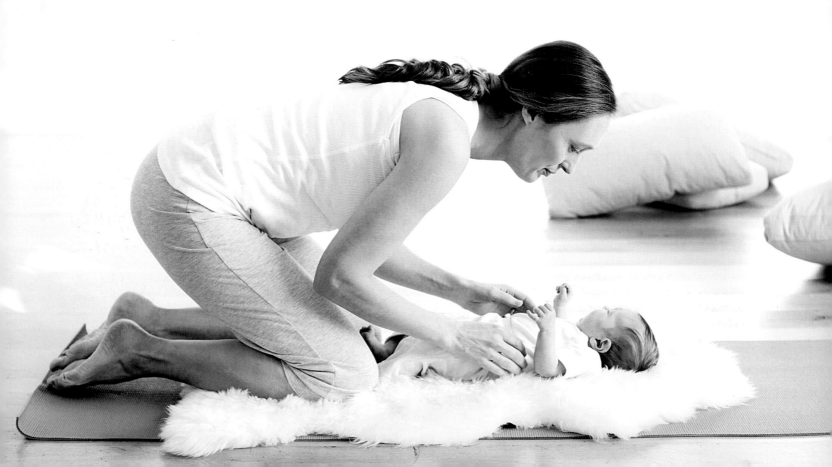

"Hello" strokes

These dry massage movements with your baby dressed will warm her up before yoga, stimulate blood flow and invite stretching in contrast with a "cradling" mode. Whichever position you adopt, either kneeling or sitting, "hello strokes" also invite you to stretch and extend your arms to prepare for sweeping, energetic yet light strokes along your baby's whole body. Greeting your baby, saying "hello" and her name, begins a special time in which she knows you are concentrating totally on her.

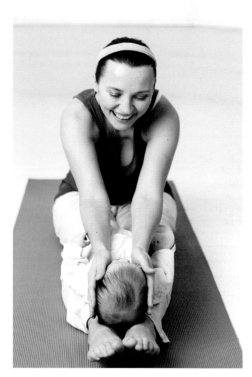 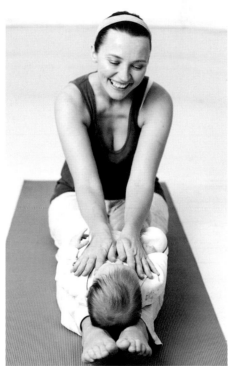 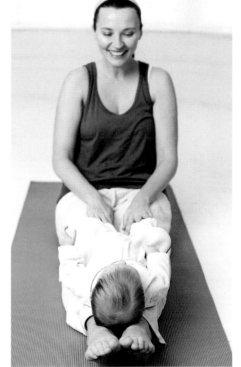

Take a breath, reach out to place both your hands on the sides of your baby's head and glide them down to her chest and along her legs, holding her feet briefly at the end of the stroke. Repeat three times.

Variation

If your baby dislikes having her head touched, start the stroke from her shoulders.

You can also say "hello" to your baby's back by gliding your hands along the sides of her body down toward her buttocks and her legs. Avoid lifting up her buttocks in this sweeping down stroke.

First hip sequence

This is the foundation of baby yoga, and indeed of yoga postures that aim at toning the deeper muscles of the body with beneficial effects on the nervous and endocrine systems.

The base of the spine is of the utmost importance in how strong, balanced, centered, and supple we are, how fully and freely we inhabit our bodies. Some babies are very supple to the point of hyper-mobility while others are surprisingly stiff. Baby yoga aims to achieve a midway balance, increasing either steadiness or suppleness.

It is important never to force any movement on your baby but always to be led by her ability at that moment. Baby yoga also helps to improve symmetry, particularly with hip movements, while respecting the limits of your baby's range of motion on each side.

Try to be aware of your breathing so that you establish a rhythm with your breath in each of the practices below.

For young or sensitive babies, start with moves 1-2-3-6-7, gradually introducing 4 and 5. For babies with clicky hips, spend longer on moves 6 and 7.

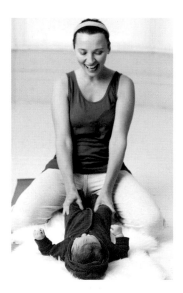

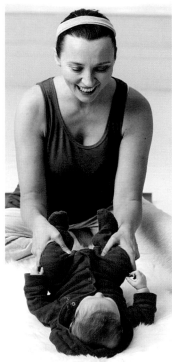

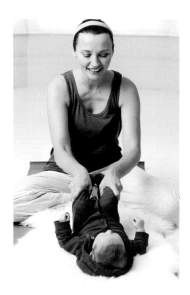

1 Check your baby's "yes" cues (page 14), placing both your hands on her legs below her knees and making eye contact.

2 Placing your hands on your baby's bent legs, and avoiding direct pressure on her knees, bring her thighs firmly toward her abdomen. Release and repeat two or three times, adjusting the pressure to suit your baby. Babies can receive, and enjoy, quite strong pressure safely, but stop at once if your baby is not happy. Alternating pressure and release stimulates your baby's digestion and relieves constipation.

3 Keeping your hands in the same position on her shins, move your baby's bent legs gently in a small circle, first clockwise, then counter-clockwise. This is your baby's first yoga twist. Make sure that you do not lift her bottom off the mat in this movement.

4 Continue by moving your baby's legs alternately toward her body and toward you in a slow pedaling action that you can make faster as she gets used to this practice.

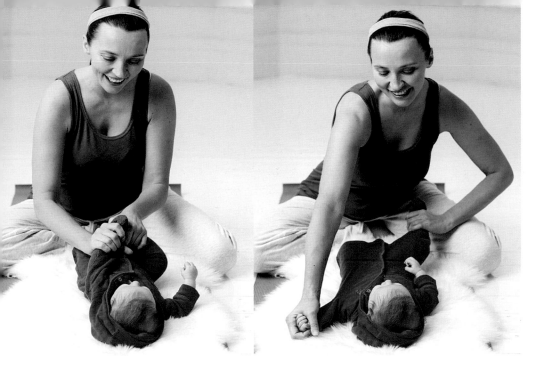

5 The diagonal stretch includes two phases. First, bring your baby's foot toward her opposite hand. Release and repeat with the other leg and hand. Never force hand and foot to touch if they don't do so easily.

The second phase is a diagonal stretch of your baby's arm and leg away from her body. Be tentative at first. Babies love this movement once they are happy to stretch their arms away from their chests, but for some, particularly babies born prematurely, it may take a little while to gain enough trust to do this.

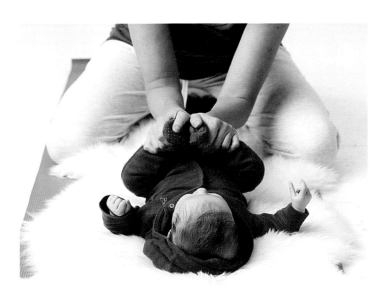

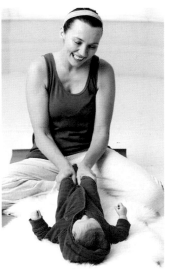

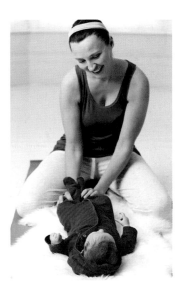

6 Just as in the classic yoga butterfly pose, this prepares your baby's hip joints for movement while also toning the lower back muscles. Hold her lower legs with your thumbs under her heels and your fingers around the ankles, and bring the soles of her feet together. Gentle tap-taps of the feet—ideally while you are talking or singing to her—add fun to this pose. Once your baby is familiar with the butterfly position, you can press her feet gently toward her tummy and release for a stronger action.

7 From butterfly, bring your baby's legs together and draw her knees slightly inward in a counterpose to the previous move. Repeat three times. This is a soothing, rhythmical way to bring the first hip sequence to a close.

8 Relax your baby by holding her feet for a few seconds.

Hip sequence — more moves

These movements make the first hip sequence more interactive, eliciting responses from your baby. Once he is familiar with the first sequence, integrate extra steps one by one. Babies enjoy novelty most if it fits within an established routine. After their third month, they will let you know clearly what they like.

Body twist (add to Step 3)

Change your hold of your baby's legs so that your fingers are around and your thumb under each leg. Extend one leg over the other. Keep his hip as close to the mat as possible. This is a wonderful help for your baby to integrate postural reflexes as he develops at his own pace.

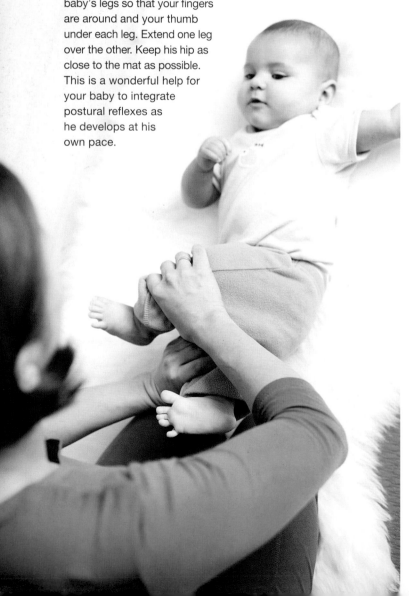

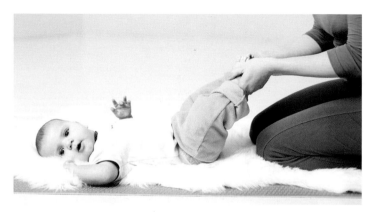

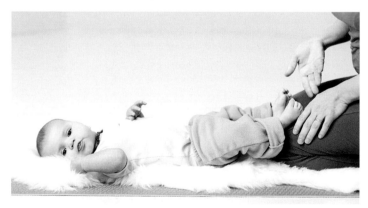

Lift, drop, relax (add to Step 7)

Babies love safe surprises. They learn opposites with their bodies long before they can grasp them conceptually. Here is a first pair of opposites you can introduce. Holding your baby's ankles loosely, lift his legs and release your hold at once in order to let them flop. Repeat three times. You can say the words "stretch" and "relax" with each action. This is a relaxing way to end an active hip sequence, and also a practice you can use to calm a baby who kicks his feet in the air frantically or arches his back when upset.

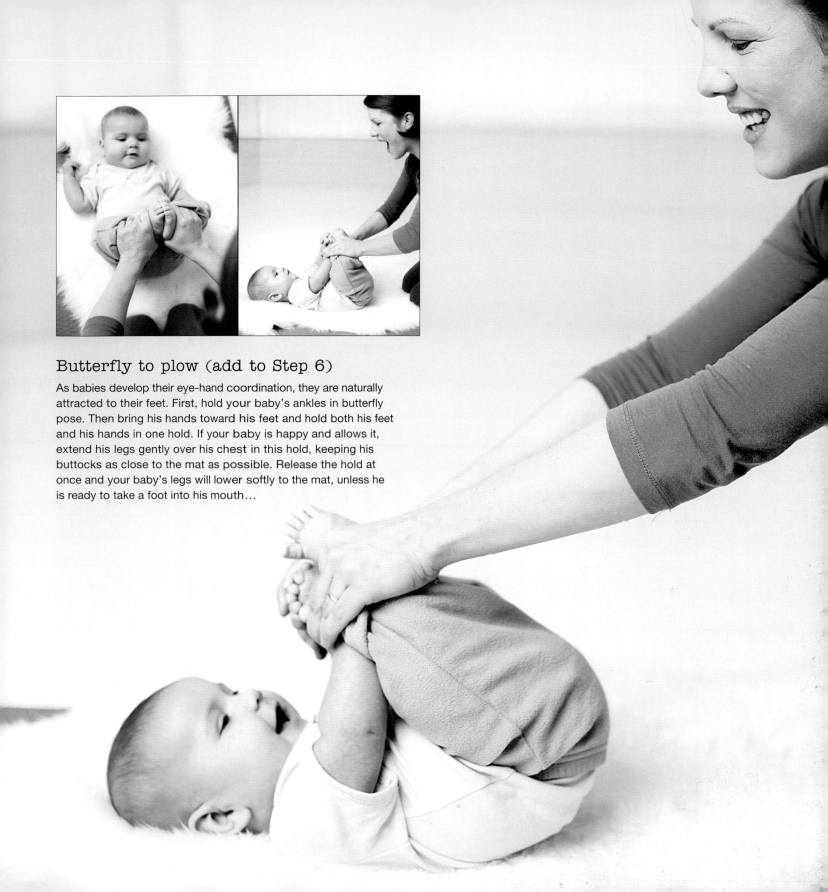

Butterfly to plow (add to Step 6)

As babies develop their eye-hand coordination, they are naturally attracted to their feet. First, hold your baby's ankles in butterfly pose. Then bring his hands toward his feet and hold both his feet and his hands in one hold. If your baby is happy and allows it, extend his legs gently over his chest in this hold, keeping his buttocks as close to the mat as possible. Release the hold at once and your baby's legs will lower softly to the mat, unless he is ready to take a foot into his mouth…

Prone hip sequence

This sequence makes "tummy time" enjoyable for your baby through a variety of activities combining dry massage and yoga. If sitting on a mat is not comfortable for you, sit on a bed or couch with your back supported. You cannot check how receptive your baby is by making eye contact in this position, but she will either show you a relaxed back or try to squirm out of it. If the latter is the case, pick her up gently and stroke her back while carrying her in shoulder hold (page 19.) Leave it a couple of days before trying again.

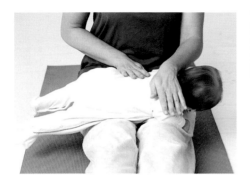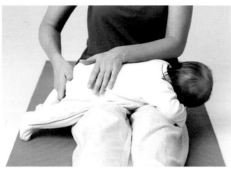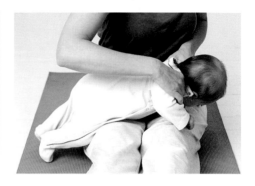

1 Place your baby on her front across your thighs. Make sure that her upper chest rests well on your thigh so that her head is supported, whether or not she has gained head control. Rub your hands across her back from shoulders to buttocks with to and fro strokes. Glide your hands back to the top and repeat twice more, always avoiding any direct pressure on her spine.

2 Holding one hand against your baby's buttocks, slightly cup your other hand in order to avoid pressure on her spine, and massage your baby's lower back down toward her buttocks. Press your hands gently toward each other, hold for a moment, then release.

3 Place the fingertips of both your hands on each side of your baby's neck, then lift and flutter them down your baby's back like the pitter patter of raindrops. Adjust the tempo and intensity to your baby's liking and end with a couple of long slow strokes down her back.

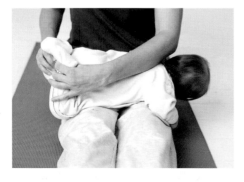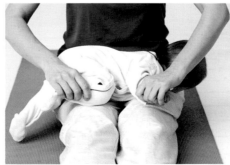

4 Continue with gentle leg stretches. Hold your baby's ankles with your thumbs over and your fingers under her legs. Bring her feet together close to her buttocks as in butterfly (page 39), then release.

5 If your baby is ready for more, hold her far ankle and wrist. Then bring her elbow and knee toward each other, and release. Repeat three times, allowing full release of the limbs.

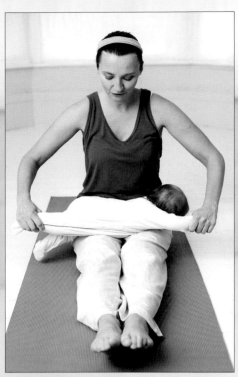

6 Hold your baby's ankle and wrist on the side that is farther away from you, with your fingers on the outer part of her limbs. Gently extend her arm and leg into a stretch that is comfortable for her. She will make it clear to you with her body response whether she enjoys a greater or lesser stretch. Never force. Do this stretch once and release fully.

7 Holding your baby's head and feet in each hand at the end of this sequence is soothing and relaxing. It can also be healing if your baby had a long and difficult birth.

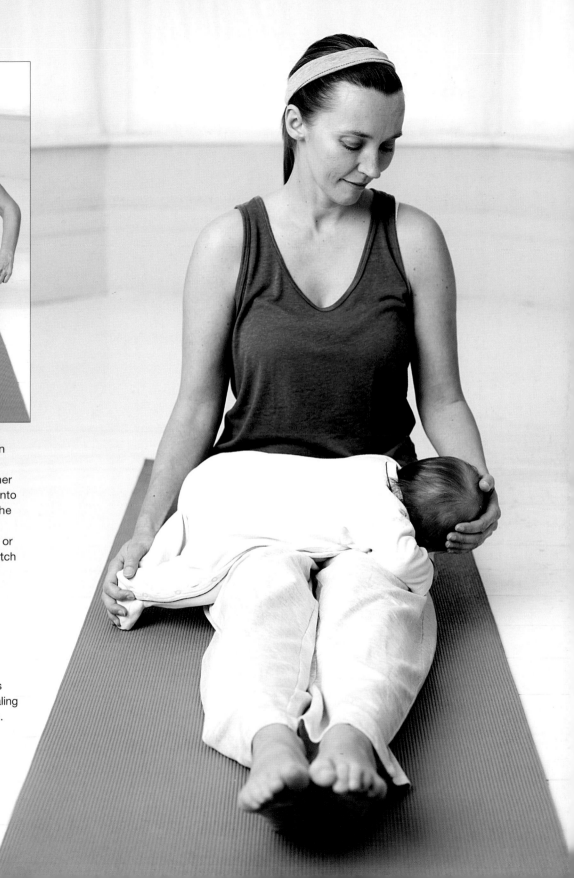

Cradle rolls to rolling baby

Not just rocking but also rolling are required for healthy brain development, particularly the part of the brain that is responsible for how we orient ourselves in space and learn to balance. Your baby will have done a lot of rolling inside the womb, as long as there was space to do so, and within just a few weeks after birth, she can progress from tiny rolls in cradle hold to an adventurous rolling journey down your legs and back again. How and when this happens depends mainly on how safe your baby feels. Each baby is different and the art of baby yoga is to offer just the stimulation your baby needs at any particular time—no less, but no more either.

Watch your baby's response carefully as you progress from tiny to larger movements. If you go too far and your baby becomes distressed, return to a more familiar practice for a few days and wait for her lead to do more.

Cradle rolls

1 Quarter roll

Adapt cradle hold (page 18) by encircling your baby's arm gently but securely with your upper hand and extending your lower arm through her legs. Roll her carefully to face outward and roll her back. This small movement is welcomed by even the most sensitive babies.

2 Half roll

From the adapted cradle hold, roll your baby out with a quarter roll and then roll her back toward you by lifting the elbow that supports your baby's head. This is the first baby yoga move that alternates moving away from you, away from home, and then returning home to be close to you. This rolling game can be a source of security to your baby because each time she is rolled back she can focus on your face, and is happy to find you there again.

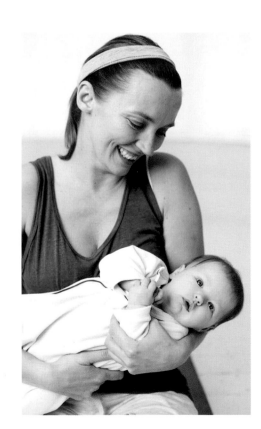

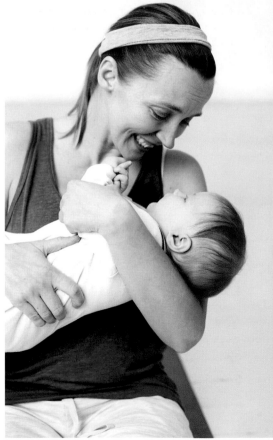

Roll and gentle drop

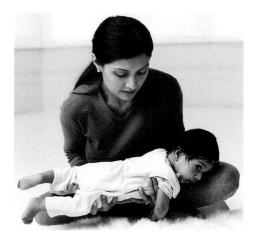

2 Lowering your hands and lifting your elbows slightly makes your baby roll over away from you. Release your hands as he rolls and drops. His body will be relaxed, which is something all mammal babies are programed to do. Babies are usually surprised by the sensation, but delighted. This is an excellent preparation for spontaneous rolls to come, and is also reassuring for babies who are easily startled.

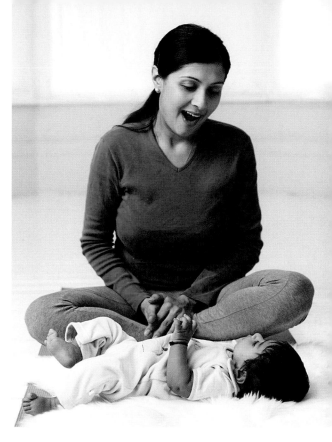

1 From a "tummy time" position, lying face down across your legs, lift your baby gently by placing your forearms under his upper chest and his hips, half an inch or so from a soft rug or blanket.

Rolling baby

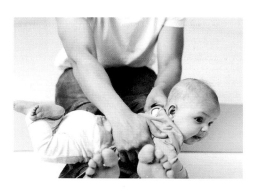 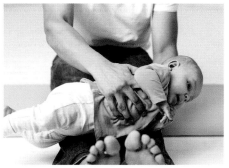 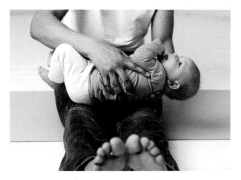

1 In order to roll your baby down your legs and back again, she must have gained head control. It is therefore preferable to wait until your baby is able to raise her head confidently when lying on her front.

2 Your baby's comfort in the rolls depends on the combination of your hand movements—one hand stabilizes the shoulder that rolls while the other hand moves her hip in the roll. The better synchronized these two actions become, the easier it is for your baby to roll smoothly down your legs and back again.

3 Start with one full roll from your thighs to your shins before attempting further rolls either toward your body or further down toward your feet. Your technique and your baby's technique develop together. Dads are usually keen and often excel at "rolling baby."

Up and down with your baby

While your baby is still small and light, it is important to acquire positive habits so that you can pick him up and lower him into a crib or to the floor without straining your back. Aligned and harmonious movements not only make life with your baby more enjoyable from day to day, they are also important in helping him develop body awareness, confidence, and agility.

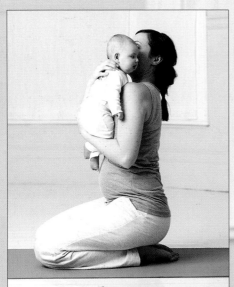

Hug up, hug down

You can make use of shoulder hold to pick up and lower your baby smoothly. It is easiest to practice this movement from a kneeling position on a mat. Slide your stronger hand under your baby's bottom and your other hand under the base of her head. Bring her to your chest in an upright shoulder hold, heart to heart. Taking a moment to synchronize your heart beats before putting her down to sleep can make all the difference. Your baby will love the sensation and associate it with closeness to you. When lowering your baby from shoulder hold, move slowly and gently. Talking to her and smiling makes it easier for her to fall asleep happily after you leave.

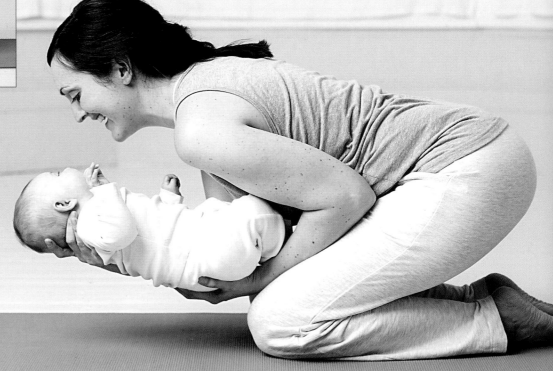

Scoop turn around

Millions of parents around the world pick up their new babies from the
floor in this way from their third month to their third year.

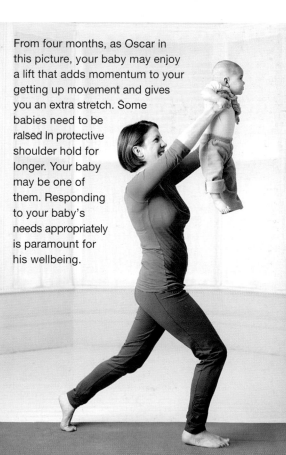

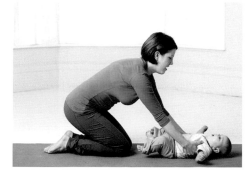

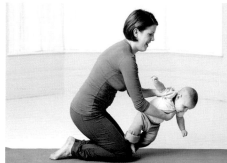

1 From a kneeling position, slide your
stronger hand under your baby's upper
back and extend your other hand to hold
his upper arm safely between your thumb
and index finger.

2 Use the hand under your baby's upper back to roll his chest onto your banister arm
and then lift him to your chest facing away from you. With a little practice this becomes a
swift scoop and turn around that you can use in reverse to roll your baby to the floor.

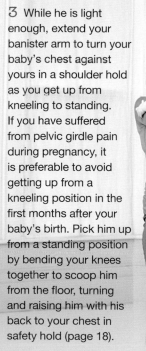

3 While he is light
enough, extend your
banister arm to turn your
baby's chest against
yours in a shoulder hold
as you get up from
kneeling to standing.
If you have suffered
from pelvic girdle pain
during pregnancy, it
is preferable to avoid
getting up from a
kneeling position in the
first months after your
baby's birth. Pick him up
from a standing position
by bending your knees
together to scoop him
from the floor, turning
and raising him with his
back to your chest in
safety hold (page 18).

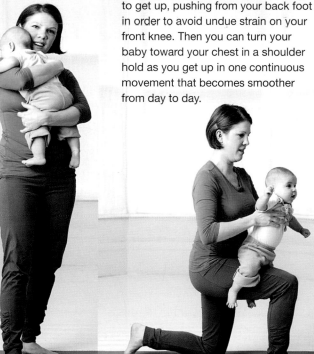

4 As your baby gets heavier, sit him
on one of your knees to make it easier
to get up, pushing from your back foot
in order to avoid undue strain on your
front knee. Then you can turn your
baby toward your chest in a shoulder
hold as you get up in one continuous
movement that becomes smoother
from day to day.

From four months, as Oscar in
this picture, your baby may enjoy
a lift that adds momentum to your
getting up movement and gives
you an extra stretch. Some
babies need to be
raised in protective
shoulder hold for
longer. Your baby
may be one of
them. Responding
to your baby's
needs appropriately
is paramount for
his wellbeing.

Mini-swings and drops

All babies like and need swings and drops. It is part of our heritage. Human babies have been carried by their mothers or siblings walking on rough terrain for thousands of years. In order to replicate the basic moves that we now know are so beneficial to brain development, baby yoga offers a safe progression starting with contained swings and drops that are first produced very gently by parents' bodies while holding their newborns. Gradually, as babies gain head control and strength, they can be held farther away.

Contained cradle swing

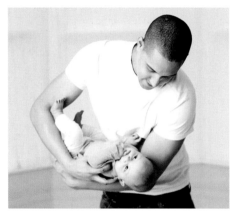

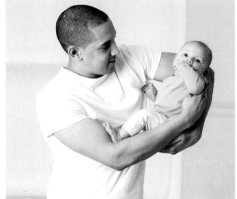

The security of a cradle hold allows a young baby to swing safely in her father's arms. Start with very small horizontal movements, watching your baby's reactions. If she is startled, extending her arms up in the air, stop and cuddle her. If she has a self-calming response to the new situation, like Daisy here with her fingers in front of her mouth, she may need a few gentle practices before relaxing into the moves.

Open cradle swing

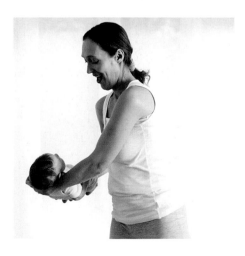

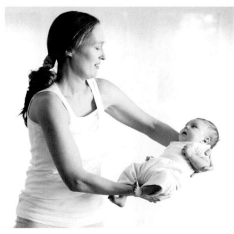

Once your baby visibly enjoys contained cradle swings, you can start opening the cradle into a semicircular movement away from your body. By placing your body weight alternately on one leg and then on the other in this wide swinging movement, you create a rhythm that is exciting and enjoyable for your baby while being able to retain eye contact throughout. At any time you can bring your baby close to your body again and recreate a cradle by sliding her head onto your relaxed elbow and supporting her lower back with your other arm.

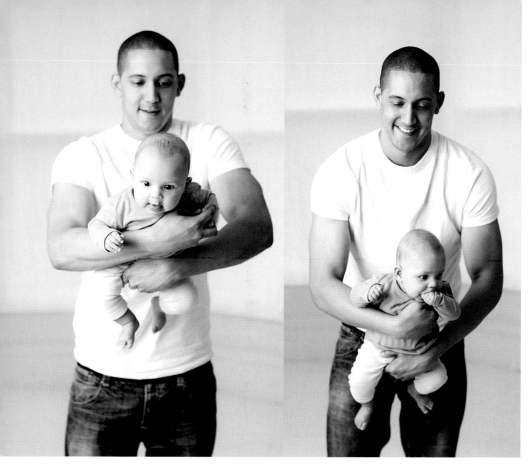

Mini-drops

With your baby's back against your chest in a safety hold, first bend your knees so that she can experience a drop by proxy without her body changing position in your arms. Very young babies find drops enjoyable and calming. Walking with babies in a safety hold and occasionally offering mini-drops coupled with deep exhalations is one way of soothing colicky babies. Repeated mini-drops is a widespread technique for calming upset babies in many parts of the world—parents must ensure that young babies' heads are kept steady and their bodies are well aligned and supported as they bend their knees for the drops.

The next step is to lower your baby down your chest so that she experiences a drop herself. With some practice this becomes a favorite for most babies.

Drop, swing, lift

Use the safety hold with your strong hand supporting your baby's seat and your banister arm extending across her chest. Clasp her upper arm securely. With this hold you can gently swing your baby forward and back. Progress gradually from small horizontal movements to longer, higher ones. Parents in Birthlight classes have given this practice the name "whooshing," and babies love to be "whooshed" toward a familiar adult or another baby. Whooshing is a foolproof way to lift your baby's mood. If you are on your own at home, you can whoosh your baby toward a mirror—seeing her happy face may cheer you up too, if you need cheering.

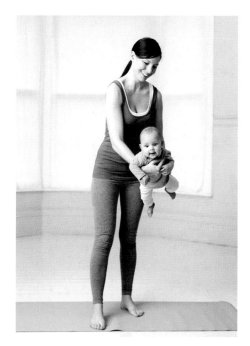
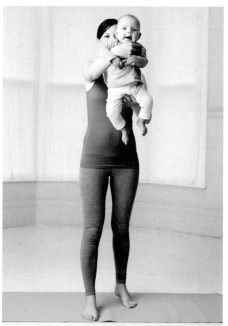

Family yoga with a young baby

Baby yoga offers a structured focus that can allow babies to experience different qualities of touch and handling from those associated with everyday care. Even with a newborn, a multitude of family scenarios are possible. Through them, all participants learn new ways of relating not just to the new baby but also to one another, sometimes discovering previously unseen qualities that the baby's presence brings out. These interactive moments can serve as relaxation. Classic relaxation, however, is the preferred completion of any yoga practice. Taking a few minutes to prepare for each day with a new baby, and to recharge, is an essential postnatal yoga practice that benefits both mother and baby.

Babies' innocent happiness at feeling valued radiates to the whole family, so celebrate small achievements with unconditional love. Although this book is mainly written for mothers, parenting roles can be shared in as many combinations as there are families.

Involving an older child with a new baby in your massage and yoga practice is not always easy. It is natural for a toddler to feel displaced and to require more attention just when you would like to give your newborn a massage. Offering a small soft doll to your toddler is a possible solution. You may find that he has already observed how you change and clean the baby, and that he is ready to learn baby massage, too. Watch him reproduce your gestures!

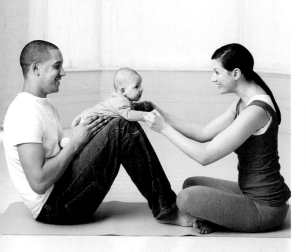

Re-encountering your baby after she has had "tummy time" on her father's lap can be like meeting her anew. The sight of your bright-eyed baby, proudly lifting her head, is exciting.

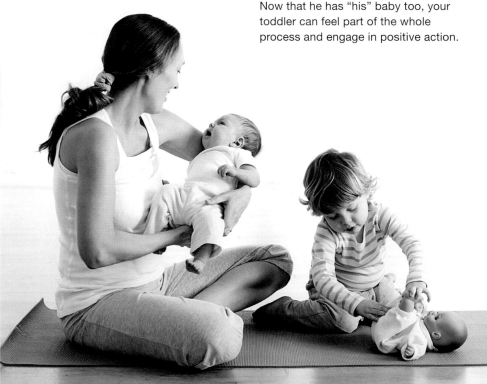

Now that he has "his" baby too, your toddler can feel part of the whole process and engage in positive action.

Relaxation with your baby

Lie down on a rug or blanket in a comfortable position. You may find it more comfortable to bend your knees for the first months. Become aware of all your "what if" concerns—perhaps set an alarm for ten minutes' time in case you fall asleep, if this worries you. Dare to close your eyes and look inward and you will realize how much all your senses have become attuned to the care of your baby—watching, listening, pacifying, adjusting. Start releasing this accumulated tension with a few deep exhalations. Voice them into sighs if this feels good. Surrender to being here, right now, with no agenda. Let your mind know that you are away on a little vacation. Tasks and thoughts can wait. Whether or not this is your first baby, so much has changed in your life and you need to keep connected with your true self. Your unconscious is better at helping you do this in relaxation than while you sleep. Several techniques can help new mothers relax with their babies, first of all while the baby is sleeping.

Nurturing yourself

Acknowledge any emotions associated with your baby's birth. If you feel the need for healing, decide to do something about it in the near future. Then recall with wonder that your baby is here, close to you. Let the awareness of what you need to nurture yourself surface from your unconscious. Do not discard anything that comes to you, as trivial as it may seem. Relax the palms of your hands so they are soft and you can fully receive and fully give all around.

Where do you store your baby's crying? Feel where the crying goes. It may be in your chest but also in your neck, your lower back, even your calf muscles.

Focus your attention on your breathing. First allow yourself to yawn as you exhale. Then hum steadily through three exhalations. Relax your jaw and absorb yourself in this soothing resonance. Once you are familiar with this practice, try relaxing with your baby after feeds and gradually at any time either of you needs a little time out.

After a few tries your baby will start synchronizing with your relaxation. Each joint relaxation gives you greater awareness of how you and your baby respond to each other's moods and of the calming power of your breathing.

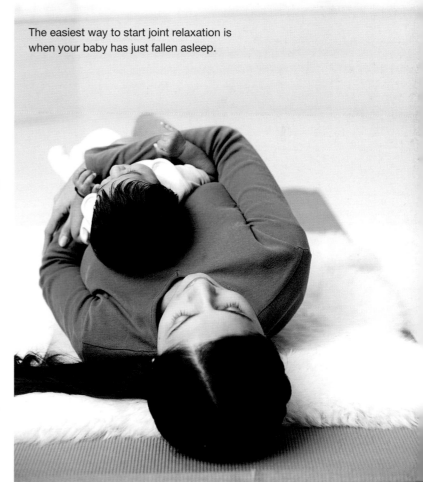

The easiest way to start joint relaxation is when your baby has just fallen asleep.

3 Baby Yoga after Four Months

During the fifth month, babies tend to become more aware of their bodies and themselves in relation to parents and surroundings. A four-month-old baby loves communicating through active play and starts to try to copy what he observes, often vocalizing his delight, especially when talked or sung to. Using his head control to the full, he is able to explore rolling, and to increase his strength through short pull-ups and sit-ups that give him both immense pleasure and frustration. With your relaxing and toning massage routine now established, or easier to introduce at this stage, this is the ideal time to expand baby yoga in a more dynamic way. Practices in this chapter help you support your growing baby's desire to engage with the world while retaining the safety of your arms and the closeness of your body.

Add pressure and movement

If you have already massaged your baby and done yoga with him, you may have noticed how the range of his responses has changed. Whether he likes energetic swings and lifts or prefers long cuddly relaxations, enjoys being massaged on his back or already loves wriggling and rolling away, he seeks to be more and more involved in the activities that he enjoys. You, his mother, continue to fascinate him and he starts inviting you to play new games of communication and action.

In this chapter, familiar stretches are expanded to match your baby's greater confidence and strength, while some are introduced for the first time. With more definite and diverse rhythms, you can show him clearer contrasts between activity and rest. Yoga moves and relaxation in combination help him to be more active when awake and to sleep more deeply. If he needs to continue with a gentler practice, include the new steps in a style that suits him. Assisting without ever forcing, whether physically or through conditioning, remains the golden rule of baby yoga at this stage.

In responding to your baby's clearer "yes, more" or "no, not this, not now," you need to be resourceful. The negotiation of boundaries is already starting. Baby massage and yoga can help set foundations of mutual accommodation that can last a lifetime. Respecting your baby's individuality is essential but so is your centering and firmness. As much as tender love, your baby now requires your active support and guidance.

Pay greater attention to your breathing in energetic moves. This is the way to teach your baby effortless use of the breath in movement as a life skill.

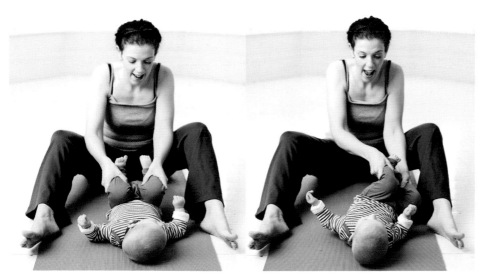

Introduce a stronger contrast between pressure and release in knees to chest, and a greater and speedier flexion of your baby's legs to involve his whole spine in knee circles.

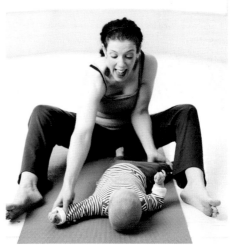

Add a more definite extension of your baby's arm and leg in diagonal stretch.

Dynamic hip sequence

Babies over four months strive to stretch out to gain the strength that will free their movement later on. This more dynamic hip sequence safely promotes maximum flexibility of the pelvic joints while extending and relaxing all the lower back and abdominal muscles.

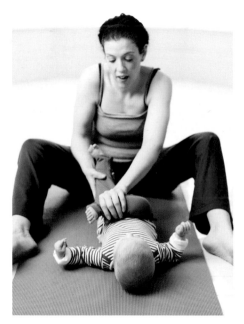 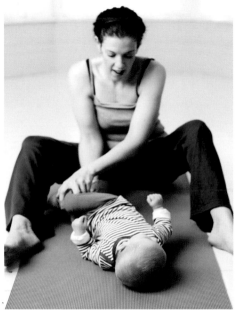 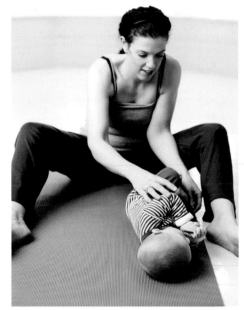

1 Half lotus

This is an asymmetrical movement of your baby's legs that increases hip suppleness. Hold one of his lower legs with your fingers over the leg and thumb under it. Bring his foot over the opposite hip (this is a half-lotus position.) At the same time, hold his other leg extended along the mat, encouraging a full stretch if possible. Your baby may progress to an acrobatic half lotus by extending his foot toward the opposite armpit, and even as far as touching his nose. It is important that your baby leads this progression. Release your hold if you feel any resistance.

2 Twist and roll to the side

Beyond a full body twist (page 40), you can now encourage your baby to roll over on his side. This will be well received if he is already attempting to roll by himself, otherwise you may prefer to wait. Add greater momentum in the twist by crossing your arms over while twisting your baby alternately to one side and then the other. He may need a little additional support under either his hip or his shoulder in order to get the satisfaction of rolling.

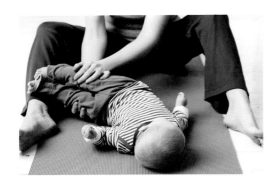

3 Extended leg twist

Your baby may now enjoy a supine body twist with his legs extended rather than flexed. Hold his legs firmly with both of your hands just above his knees. Inhale as you lift your baby's extended legs, exhale as you lower them to one side. Let him bend his legs if he prefers it, and keep your baby's spine on the mat the whole time throughout this movement.

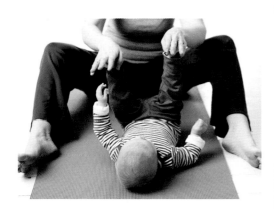

4 Push-counterpush to plow

Encourage your baby to straighten his legs by pressing a little more firmly than before on his upraised feet, giving him something to push against. This strengthens his lower back. A gentle extension of his legs over his body is then an ideal preparation for the classic plow pose. Afterward, allow your baby's whole body to unroll freely to the mat and relax for a few seconds. It is still best at this stage to keep his lower spine close to the mat as you extend his legs. Wait until he can sit up before showing him the full plow pose with his lower back raised from the mat.

5 Finger lift

Place your index fingers in your baby's hands while he is lying down on his back facing you. Let him find his own strength to raise himself up rather than you lifting him up by the arms. The movement is prompted by you but controlled by your baby. If he is not ready to raise himself fully, gently let him go down to the mat with your fingers still in his hands. Try again after a few days.

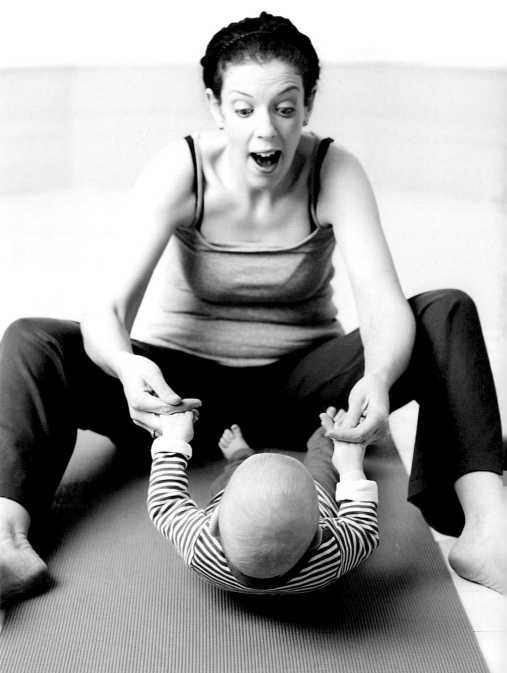

Sitting dynamic hip sequence

Introduce your baby to this sequence once she shows how much she enjoys being upright. You may choose to sit her on your lap or on the floor between your legs, but she will need your body as a back support even after she has started sitting independently. End the sequence with a game or a cuddle.

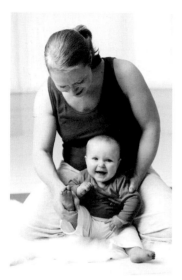 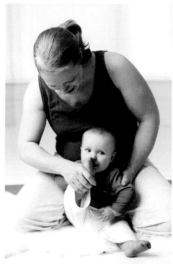

1 Leg out stretch

Help your baby gain strength and flexibility by raising alternate legs from a sitting position. Support her under one armpit so that she does not roll sideways, grasp her ankle on the other side and raise her leg outward. Do not try to extend her leg at this stage. This is a base for half lotus and knee to chest followed by a leg extension. Repeat twice on both sides.

2 Toes to nose

This time raise her leg more centrally. Bringing toes to nose delights most babies at this stage. Small ankle rotations can complement the move. Do not force her leg to go that far if she is still stiff. Regular practice of leg lifts makes this move accessible to most babies.

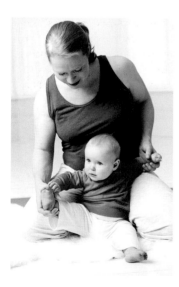 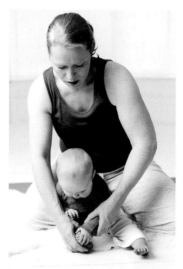

3 Diagonal sitting stretch and forward bend

Repeat Step 1 but rather than holding her under the armpit, hold her wrist on the arm opposite the raised leg. Stretch out both her arm and leg diagonally in an extended body twist. She may spontaneously reach out toward her raised foot, in line with her extended arm. In a steady rhythm, inhale as you extend your baby's arm and leg and as you exhale, lower her raised leg to the floor, returning her extended arm forward to reach her foot in a diagonal forward bend. Alternate this diagonal stretch and forward bend three times on each side, with awareness of your breathing rhythm.

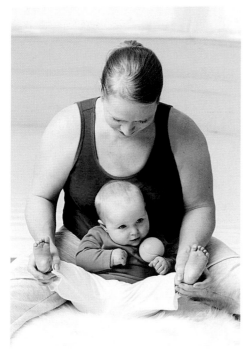
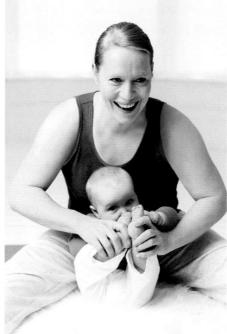
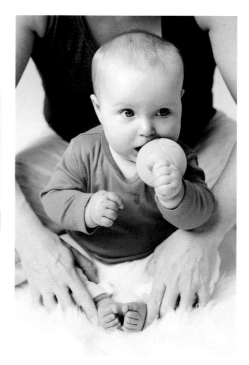

5 Open V

Holding your baby in sitting baby butterfly, lift both of her legs out to the sides, stretching them if she lets you. You will need to lean forward a little to support her back as this action tends to make babies roll back. Alternate opening out your baby's legs and bringing them back together again, tapping her feet.

6 Sitting balance with legs up

This is an extension of toes to nose, taking both feet up at the same time in a supported sitting balance that can model the classic yoga pose. Never force and leave out this pose if your baby does not enjoy it. If she does, alternate raising her legs and lowering them by simply extending your arms and leaning forward slightly yourself. If your baby is ready, you can move forward together in a joint forward bend on an exhalation. Do not hold the sitting balance for more than a few seconds.

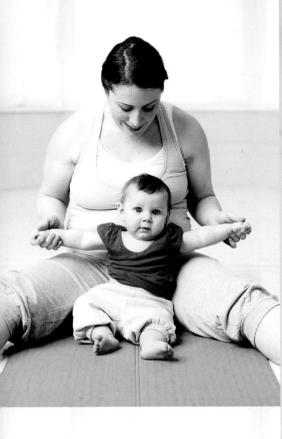

"Open and shut"

With your baby on your lap or sitting in front of you, supported by your body, use this endearing rhyme to help him stretch his arms fully. Babies who have been resisting upper body massage or dislike stretching out their arms will benefit from this especially. A gradual progression with a focus on the cuddle produces visible relaxation after a few days of practice. All babies are receptive to the loving ending of this rhyme.

"Open and shut them, open and shut them": Alternate stretching out your baby's arms as much as he allows without tension and bringing them close to his body again, holding this hands together against his chest. A slower rhythm works best for this rhyme.

"Don't get in a muddle": Hold hand over hand.

"Open and shut them, open and shut them": As before.

"Give yourself a cuddle": Cross your baby's arms on his chest and enjoy a close cuddle together.

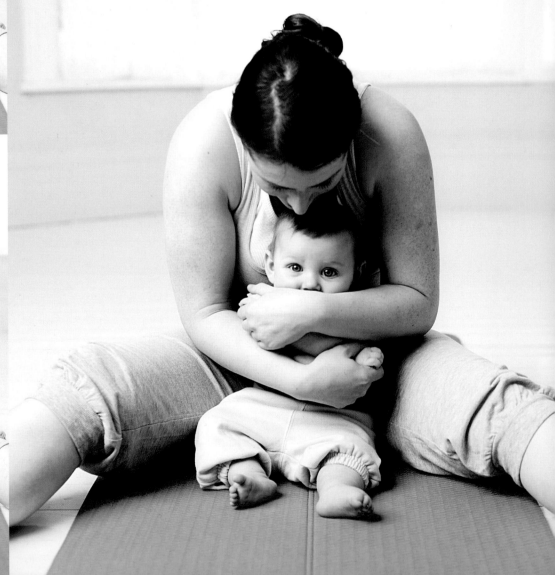

Arm openers with songs

Talking and singing to your baby are very much part of baby massage and yoga. Active rhymes combined with rhythmical movements help your baby's coordination, language, and cognitive development. Rhymes are particularly helpful with upper body stretches, which many babies resist more than leg and hip stretches. The marked contrast between stretching and relaxing movements is an ever novel source of surprise and fun that can delight your baby as an instant practice or help him forget a discomfort in a few seconds.

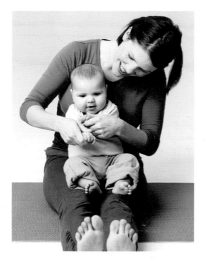
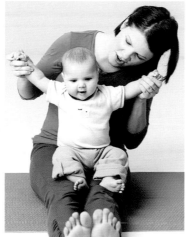

"Wind the bobbin up"

Install your baby on your lap, his back supported by your body, and combine the words and actions of this ever-popular rhyme.

"Wind the bobbin up": Hold both your baby's hands and, with a tempo that suits you both, roll one over the other outward.

"Pull, pull": Open both his arms wide to the sides.

"Clap clap clap": Clap his hands together—coordinated hand clapping comes later.

"Wind it back again": Roll his hands inward.

"Pull, pull": Open both his arms wide to the sides.

"Clap clap clap": Clap his hands together.

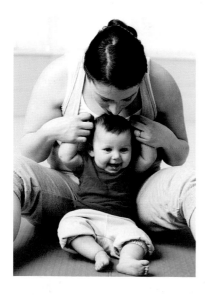
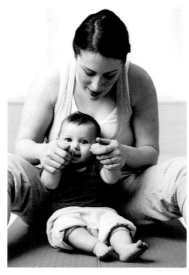

"Head, shoulders, knees, and toes"

Holding your baby's wrists, go through the motions of this popular rhyme. Not only does this help with various yoga stretches, it also helps him to gain familiarity with different parts of his body and face.

"Head, shoulders, knees and toes, knees and toes,
Head, shoulders, knees and toes, knees and toes,
Eye, mouth and ears and nose, a-and nose,
Head, shoulders, knees and toes, knees and toes."

Dynamic baby rolls

Whether or not your baby rolls over by himself just yet, it is now time to introduce a more dynamic baby rolling practice during which he can experience a range of different stretches. Rather than rolling him down and up your legs, help him to roll only at crucial points when he needs your support, and allow him time to experience new sensations and different perspectives without your interference. This is a new phase in his relationship with you. He will anticipate your actions yet enjoy his new-found freedom. Within seconds, rolls take your baby on an adventure in which you also participate.

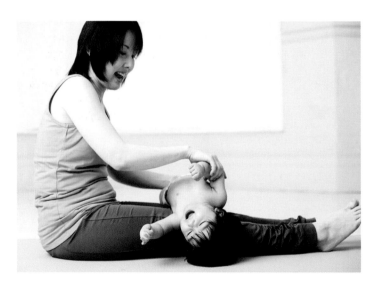

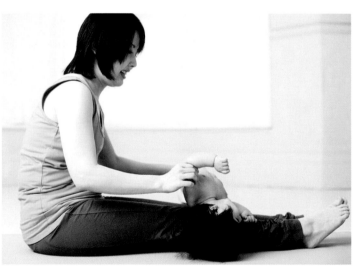

1 Back bends across your legs can be very enjoyable for babies once they relax. If your baby does not relax easily, go back to the first baby rolls (pages 44–45). Make these short rolls more dynamic, reversing and rolling forward again, alternating fast and slow motions. Play games to start and finish, ending with cuddles. Then do it again, resting your baby on his back across your legs and checking that he can relax into a back bend and "floppy rag doll" state before engaging in a full roll. He will come to understand that the more he relaxes, the easier the rolling becomes.

2 To help a baby roll after four months, a gentle tug or push of one shoulder may be sufficient. Many babies still need a complementary action of your other hand on the rolling hip. Progress gradually from a hip and arm to arm only action when your baby gains momentum in the rolls. The faster you are able to help him roll, the easier it becomes for him to do it by himself. With practice, you will develop a better synchronization with your baby's movement.

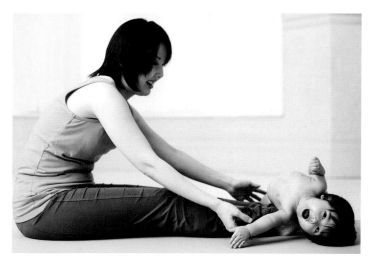

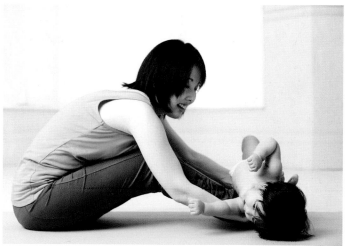

3 Your baby reaching your ankles can produce suspense. Some babies enjoy this idea of destination, and relax, others are aware of the drama. Is mummy ready to come to the rescue? Remain attentive to your baby as his emotions can shift in a split second from enjoyment to panic.

4 Communication, always part of baby yoga, is crucial when babies need to find their way. While the response with younger babies is to take them into your arms for a safe relaxed hold, now you need to assess whether your baby needs to be shown how to help himself or truly needs rescuing and comforting. Baby yoga can help you develop greater awareness of parenting options.

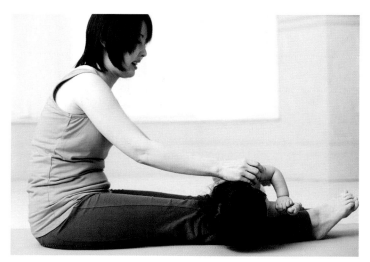

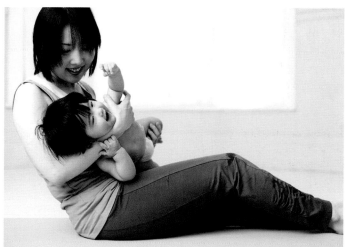

5 Make baby rolls work for you by drawing in your abdominal muscles and pelvic floor in this classic yoga sitting pose as you roll your baby back. Let him decide whether he wants to roll out again but avoid doing more than three full rolls.

6 While cuddles with younger babies at the end of a movement sequence imply home and security, as babies grow, cuddles can become a short pause while anticipating more action. Even so, they remain important for "touching home."

See-saw

Sit your baby sideways on your thighs, facing out. Support him first with an arm across his chest and then with your hands on his chest and upper back. Encourage small movements of his body, alternately releasing the hand on which he is not resting directly, and gradually allow more and more space between your hands and his body.

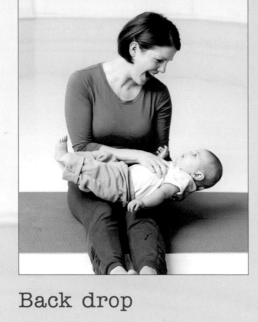

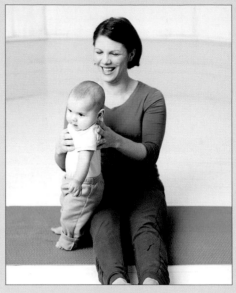

Back drop

Once your baby enjoys small movements, bend your supporting leg slightly and, reducing the support of the hand behind him, let him drop backward. Keep your hands in place so that you can catch him just when it feels right. If he is startled, throwing his arms in the air, comfort him and go back to see-saw until he can relax into a back drop.

Forward stand

Using a small lift of your other leg and a push from your back hand, create the momentum for your baby to flip back up and land in a forward stand between your hands. Many babies enjoy standing for a second or two in a supported position before they are ready to bounce on their legs. A baby who is not ready to stand up will either sit back or kneel forward. Repeat this balance three times.

Sitting balances

Balances from a sitting position encourage babies to develop good posture while coping with destabilizing movements. In classic yoga, still balances are an important way of gaining focus and stimulating the nervous system. With babies, balances are gently supported between forward and backward movements.

If your baby resists back drops, holding on to his "righting reflex," which helps him regain an upright posture after being destabilized, respect this temporary resistance and try again later when he can let go playfully. These sitting balances aim to help you slowly reduce support in a way that feels safe to your baby.

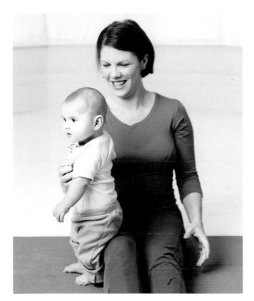 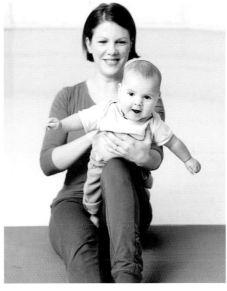 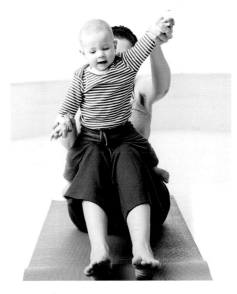

Wild ocean

If your baby giggles and is clearly happy, allow even more space between your hands. Completely release the support of your front hand when allowing him to drop back and then of your back hand as he lands upright, just resting your front hand on his chest.

Perched balance

Sitting astride one of your bent legs helps your baby to develop greater strength around the base of his spine. He has just three support points—your knee, and both of your hands, one supporting his chest and the other his back. This is an interactive balance in which pressure from either or both of your hands will help him stretch his back and the center of his body. He may hold on to your knee to start with, but gradually he will feel free to stretch his lower back, stretch out his arms and truly balance on your knee.

Arm stretches in perched balance

Once your baby has gained sufficient lower back strength, he may enjoy arm stretches while perched on one or both your knees. If he is not ready, he will not be able to maintain his balance—lower your legs to the floor in a fun drop while holding his arms. Clasp him around his body at first, and then hold his arms and finally his hands before stretching his arms first up and then out diagonally.

Upside down

As your baby develops, the "tummy time" you offer him needs to be more varied and fun with back stretches. The roller-coaster ride offers you both a fair deal of exercise and enjoyment, and leads on to your baby's first inversions. Holding a baby upside down looks dramatic but it is actually quite safe. In fact, most babies love being upside down. Just follow simple guidelines.

Roller-coaster

Front balances are an ideal foundation for your baby's first inversions. Turn your legs into a roller-coaster for rides that can be as hair-raising or gentle as he likes.

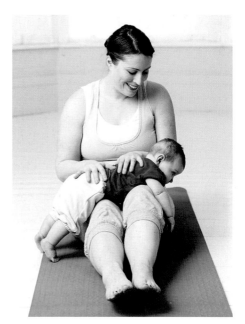

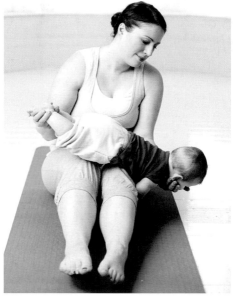

2 When you both feel ready, bend your leg under your baby's legs while holding his ankles firmly. As you raise your bent leg a little higher, bring your other hand under his chin for added protection. This is an extremely safe preparation and test before you introduce inversions to your baby.

1 With your baby lying comfortably across your thighs, alternately bend one leg and stretch the other. Watch his reactions.

Caution

When bringing your baby down from inversions, first contact is with his chest. Make sure that his head and neck are protected at all times. Sit on a bed if you feel tentative at first. You will soon gain the confidence to do baby inversions on a mat.

Side inversion (hip hold)

Early inversions help to develop a sense of confidence and trust between you and your baby. They offer all the benefits of classic yoga headstands, elongating the spine, increasing blood circulation to the brain, clearing lungs, and stimulating the nervous system. Start by holding her to the side.

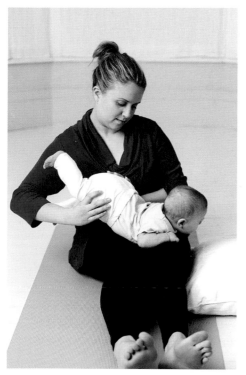 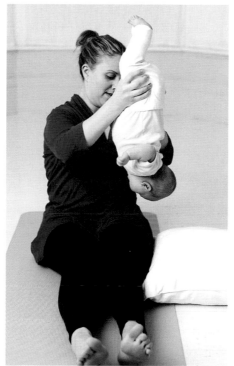 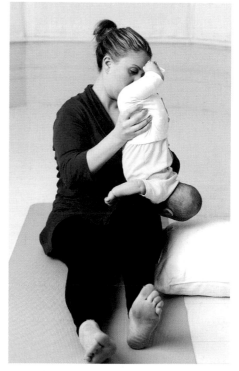

1 Place your baby on her front across your thighs with her feet to the side of your stronger hand. Make sure you place a cushion or pillow along your legs on her head side. After a few roller-coasters, slide your hands under your baby's hips and in one firm and clear movement lift her in the air to a height that is comfortable for you. You can see her face—your baby is your leader in this pose.

2 To bring her down, bend and raise your leg by the pillow so that you can rest her chest on your thigh, and lower her gently across your thighs once again. This often prompts your baby to stretch her back and lift her head to look at you. Repeat once or twice but no more.

First inversions

First baby inversions are introduced progressively with hip holds rather than holding babies from their ankles. Follow instructions carefully.

Flow inversion (hip hold)

Once you have gained confidence with side inversions, and it is clear that your baby is enjoying them, try a more dynamic flow that includes a supported full tumble for your baby. In this flow inversion, you see your baby off and greet him again but lose sight of his face when he is upside down. This is his journey! The more flowing your movement becomes, the more enjoyable it is for your baby.

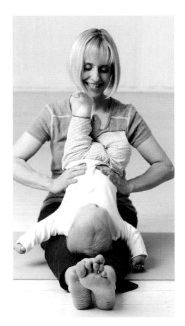 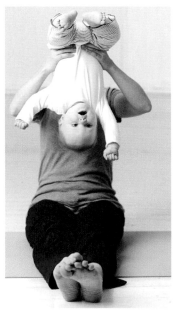 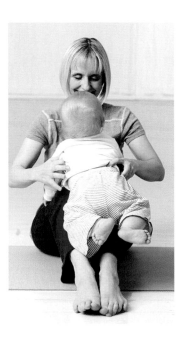 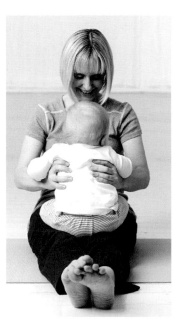

1 Sit with your legs straight out and have your baby lying on or between your legs, facing you. Take a firm hold of his hips.

2 Take a breath and, in one continuous movement, draw his body close to yours and lift him upside down.

3 At the same time bend your legs. As you exhale, gently lower your baby to rest his chest on your knees, with his head above your knees.

4 Turn your hands around on his body so that you can lift him to a sitting position on your knees and straighten your legs out again.

If your baby is ready for another loop, extend him gently on his back and repeat the flow inversion. Practice following the rhythm of your breath. Do not repeat more than three times.

Dynamic lifts

After four months most babies take delight in higher lifts but they may not be ready yet for being thrown up in the air! Held lifts are an ideal way to progress gently to these dynamic throws. Some very young babies develop a taste for them while others take it more slowly. Baby lifts are also an excellent way for you to tone your abdominal muscles, and strengthen your back—inhale as you lift and exhale as you stretch up.

From sitting

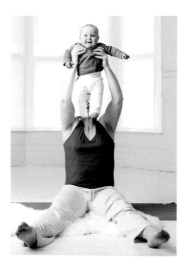

Hold your baby firmly under her arms, facing either away from or toward you. Take a breath and lift her up in the air as high as you can. Exhale and lower her to the mat slowly or fast, to her liking. You can combine this lift with a sitting balance as an action rhyme:

"Zoom zoom zoom, we're going to the moon,

five, four, three, two, one, blast off!"

From kneeling

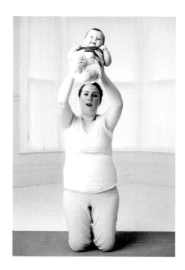

Sit on your heels with your baby on your lap facing away from you. Hold him firmly across his ribcage. Take a breath and stretch up on your knees, lifting him up in the air above your head if you can. Exhale and lower him slowly, keeping your back aligned until you are ready to sit on your heels again.

Lifting your pelvic floor muscles adds further toning for you. To make this lift more effective for you and more fun for your baby, introduce one or more stops both in the lift and in the drop, using in breaths and out breaths each time you stop.

Lift up!

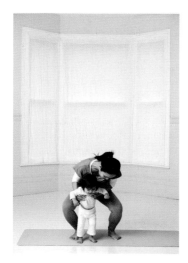 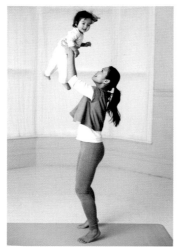

Picking up your baby from the floor, something you surely do many times each day, can also become "yoga" fun for you and your baby through body and breathing awareness. Make sure your feet are firm on the floor and you have bent your knees.

Butterfly swings

Swinging movements are a dynamic continuation of the gentle rocking that used to soothe your newborn—and are strictly for babies over four months old. Your baby will love butterfly swings and they will help her to acquire the stronger back and the balance she needs for sitting unaided. Practice them first from a kneeling position in order to protect your spinal alignment and strengthen your own back. You can also easily pick up your baby and put her down in butterfly pose.

If your baby is over four months but her seat drops well below her feet when held in butterfly pose, wait for a few weeks before starting to swing her.

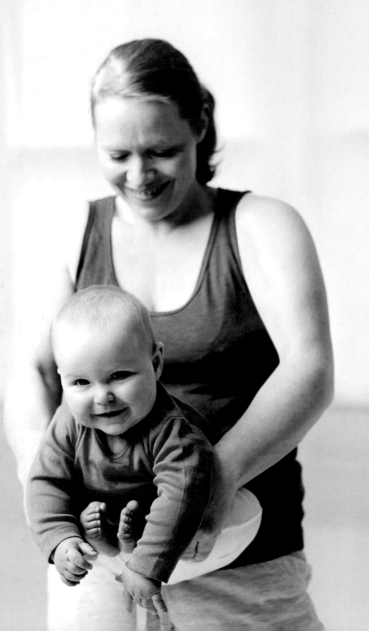

Butterfly lift from kneeling

Start from a kneeling-sitting position, as on page 56, holding your baby in butterfly pose facing away from you. Holding her ankles firmly, take a breath and kneel up, bringing her lower back against your navel area. Exhale as you lower her down to the floor again. Repeat a few times until your arms and back feel comfortable in this lift.

Sing and swing

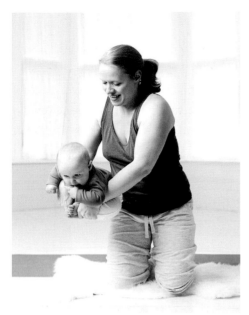

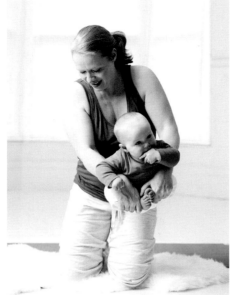

Once you have lifted your baby against your body, check that she remains aligned in butterfly pose as you move her forward slightly in front of you. Her elbows should lie relaxed on your forearms. Swing her gently at first, gradually expanding your range of movement. Let her guide you in how slow or fast, gentle or dynamic this swing needs to be today. You can add the popular rhyme "Hickory Dickery Dock" to butterfly swings, combining it with a pause against your stomach and a gentle drop.

> "Tic toc hickory dickery dock
> The mouse ran up the clock
> The clock struck one, the mouse ran down
> Hickery dickery dock, tic toc."

End with lowering your baby on to the floor in front of you, tap her feet together in a little clap and release your hold.

Butterfly lift from standing

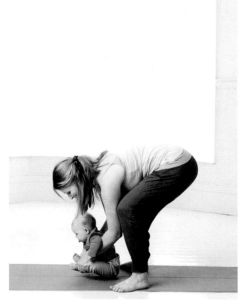

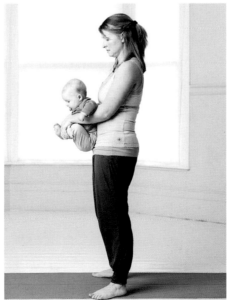

Once you have gained confidence with butterfly lifts and swings from a kneeling position, try this as a way of picking up your sitting baby from the floor. Bend your knees in a semi-squat with your feet firmly grounded. Slide your arms under her arms to bring her feet together in butterfly pose. Take a breath to lift your baby up as close to your body as possible, which is the most comfortable way. Resting her between your pubic bone and your navel can be a stable base for then sitting her on her high chair or baby seat in a neat and minimally strenuous way.

This is also a base for more dynamic butterfly swings from standing. You must ensure that your knees are slightly bent to protect your lower back, particularly as your baby is getting heavier.

Active yoga walks

These involve you and your baby in stretches that are stimulating for her, beneficial for you, and a simple way for both of you to have fun at any moment of the day, wherever you are. They integrate components of yoga and make it easier for you to start, or resume, standing poses.

They also give you greater freedom in handling your baby, enabling you to keep one hand free and teaching you to use your center of gravity to assist weight bearing with heavier babies. Many mothers all over the world use similar walks as they work and dance with their babies.

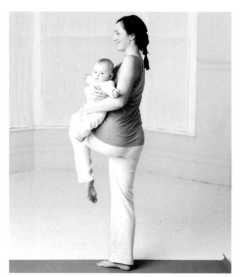

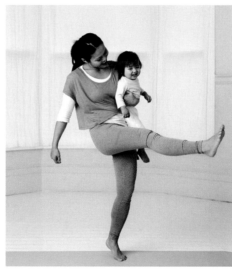

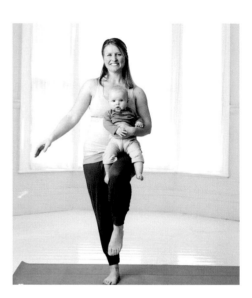

1 Walking side-twist

Start with your baby in a comfortable safety hold, facing away from you (page 18.) Lift one knee up to a height that feels easy to you and, at the same time, slide your baby onto your hip on the side of your raised leg. As you lower your leg, slide your baby to your other hip and in the flow of a stepping movement, lift your other knee. Adjust your breathing as you get into a steady rhythm. You may not go very far. This is an energetic twist in which your baby fully participates. If you feel confident, you can progress from stepping to skipping but make sure the sliding of your baby from side to side remains smooth.

2 High leg lift

As your baby gets stronger and you gain confidence with the walking side-twist, you can lift both your legs and your spirit with your baby on board. For this, you need to be confident with the safety hold using either arm, rather than both. Before you raise your leg, make sure that your baby's weight is resting on your hip bone, rather than in the hollow of your waist. This is the key to your freedom of movement, even with a heavier baby. Once your baby is in place, lift and extend your leg with gusto. Slide your baby across your body and lift your other leg.

3 Walking balance

In this walk you shift your baby from one leg to the other without taking her full weight. This is a useful skill as your baby gets heavier. Start with your baby in safety hold. Lift one knee up and slide your baby down to sit astride your thigh with her back to your body. Hold her with one arm across her chest and rest your foot on a stool or step if you need to. To change leg, bring your free arm across her chest and slide her across horizontally while lowering your raised leg and lifting your other knee. Your baby is now sitting on your other thigh. Stepping for a couple of minutes will feel like a workout.

4 Warrior walk

This adaptation of the classic warrior pose develops the walking balance with a full extension of your body while your baby rests on your front leg. Once you feel secure with your baby resting on your thigh in safety hold, step forward and stretch up your free arm. Aim at feeling a full extension from your back heel to your fingertips. Take your back foot forward in line with your front foot. Slide your baby across your body and repeat on the other side. Once you have gained confidence, step forward into an energetic walk, breathing fully in and out to create a steady rhythm.

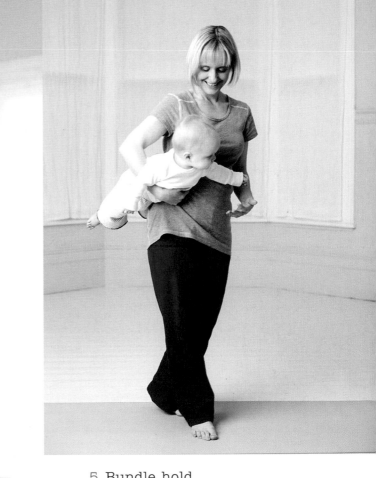

5 Bundle hold

Holding your baby face down on one side at waist level, with your forearm extending securely across his stomach, is surprisingly comfortable for both mother and baby. This hold allows you to stride, skip, and even adopt a trekking trot with your hips level and your shoulders free of tension. As your baby gets heavier, bend your knees to go uphill or downhill, upstairs or downstairs.

6 A little waltz

Active walks would not be complete without a little dance. Invite your baby for a waltz, which is most babies' favorite dancing rhythm. Hold him astride your hip, facing you, with your hand on his lower back. Holding his other hand, take off to your baby's delight.

Baby yoga before sleep

After the previous exertions, slow down, breathe more deeply with extended exhalations, and talk to your baby in a quiet voice. In this way, show your baby that it is time for sleep. Living with people who never let babies cry for more than a few seconds yet do not encounter resistance at bedtime made me realize that body language, clear intent, and awareness of babies' responses are areas in which western parents can develop finer skills to encourage their babies to fall asleep happily.

Here are a few practical suggestions that can help you shift from an active mood to a calmer one in preparation for sleep. Please note that these moves are meant as much for you as for your baby and that your state of relaxation is the most convincing basis for him to welcome your invitation to go to sleep. Developing relaxation practices will also help you to find ways to help your baby get back to sleep after waking up in the night, and possibly to wake up less.

Slow dips

These act on your baby's nervous system to make him feel sleepy. Try them first from a kneeling position.

Once you are confident, you can combine slow dips most effectively with a relaxed walk.

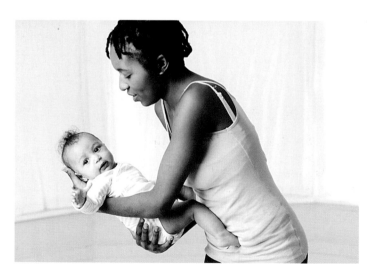

Lower your baby from shoulder hold to face you, one hand supporting his lower spine and the other his head. This support is securing for your baby at any age. If he feels heavy, bring him closer to you. Seek eye contact and tell him how sweet sleep can be.

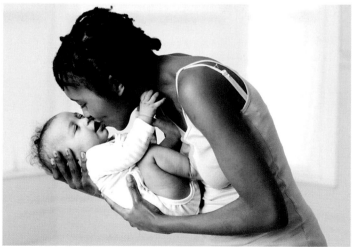

Giving your baby kisses and cuddles when you wish him to fall asleep is an ideal way to communicate to him that the world is an all right place for him to be and he can let go safely. All babies need this reassurance.

Soothing mudra and baby binding

In yoga, hand mudras are mindful gestures. They are traditionally used in India to soothe babies, and can follow a bedtime massage or be practiced on their own.

Mudras and binding holds act as playful containment, which can renew contact if you have been away from your baby, or after he has been upset or hurt.

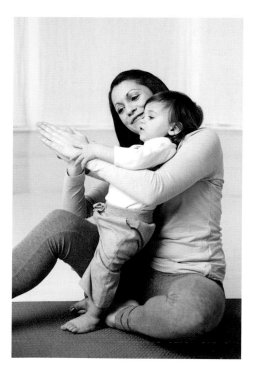

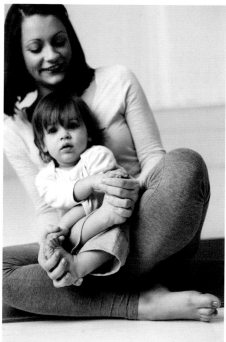

Sit with your baby on your lap or astride one of your legs against your body if he can relax in this position. Hold his hands or let him hold your wrists. Joining hands together is the most basic of all mudras. Pointing your fingers down and making snaky movements will induce calm concentration in your baby.

Sitting cross-legged or on your knees, cross your baby's arms and legs and hold hand and a foot together. Rock your baby gently from side to side in this binding hold, and sing his favorite rhyme.

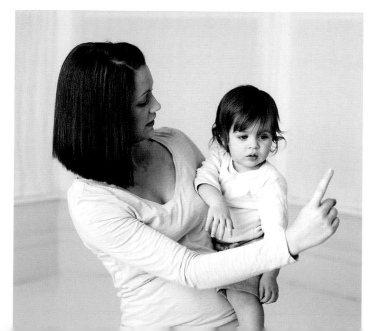

Eye tracking

Tracking objects with his gaze is calming for your baby. Simply move your index finger to the side and back to center to hold his attention. Eye tracking is most effective in combination with slow relaxed steps in the room where he is to sleep.

4 Postnatal Yoga with your Baby

Exercising with your baby is challenging at first but worth doing for both of you. The postnatal yoga practices in this chapter act directly upon your abdominal and lower back muscles, using breath and spinal moves to create deep tone. The basic stretches are easy, even if you are new to yoga, yet they are effective for all new mothers. You can integrate them with other exercises if you have already started a different program, and start them at any time irrespective of the type of birth you have experienced.

The more regularly you exercise together with your baby, the more natural this will seem to her. You will be surprised at how much she picks up long before she can move. Knowing that you can do yoga with your baby rather than excluding her from your practice also provides a useful foundation for retaining your identity without physical separation.

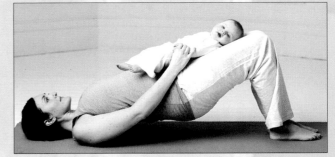

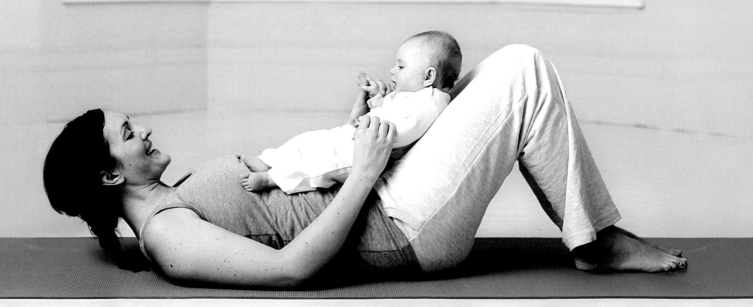

Tone your pelvic muscles

Lie down on your back with your knees bent and your feet flat at a comfortable distance from your body, not too close or too far—this is important for this exercise. Place your baby with her back on your thighs, facing you, and hold her wrists. If she is already sitting, this is fine too. There are several progressive practices you can do. As you become familiar with each of them, you will soon fit them easily in a daily round.

1 Take a breath and press your lower back toward the mat as you exhale. You are toning your abdominal muscles, drawing them toward your back muscles in this classic yoga exercise. For more intensity, press your feet down on the mat. Raise your head to look at your baby on your exhalation (see opposite) for even stronger abdominal toning. Release your neck fully, dropping your head on the mat and lifting your tailbone slightly for your next inhalation. With an even breathing rhythm, repeat six times, if your baby allows, then take a rest.

2 Once you have found a steady breathing rhythm, draw your pelvic-floor muscles inward as you inhale and continue holding them, or draw them in more, as you exhale. Release your pelvic floor at the very end of your exhalation. If you feel out of breath, inhale and exhale before starting again on the following inhalation. Feet pressure and head lift make this practice stronger. Now keep your head up through your exhalation, releasing it only at the end while you relax your pelvic floor.

3 In this practice, you tone your lower back and buttock muscles as well as your pelvic floor. Starting with your back and head flat on the floor, inhale and push from your feet to lift your lower back. Tuck in your buttock muscles and draw in your pelvic floor as you exhale. Release, lower your back to the floor and look at your baby on the next breath. With practice you can combine these exercises.

Right angle

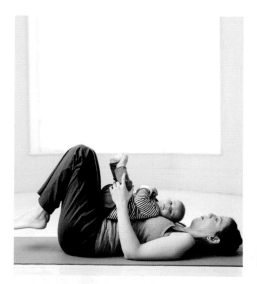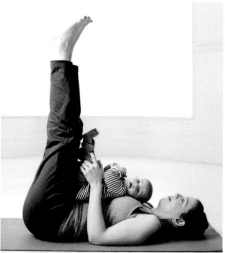

In this practice your raised legs, first bent and then straight, help you tone your abdominals and lower back with the calm power of deep breathing. Your baby can be lying on your body with his legs held up against yours. Press the base of your spine on the floor. While you are toning intensely, this pose can be very relaxing for both you and your baby, once your breathing is established enough to hold your legs up without strain. Bend your legs if they start shaking and try lifting them after a few more practices.

Baby flier

This baby yoga favorite can be a complete abdominal and back toner when done with correct spinal alignment and yoga breathing.

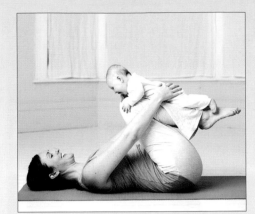

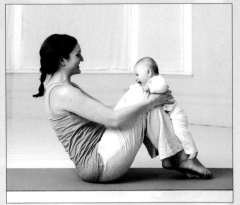

1 Lie down with your back aligned and knees bent. Have your baby facing you, either resting on your thighs or sitting. Reaching out to her, pick her up firmly under the arms and as you inhale, "fly" her forward with her face above yours. Exhale, pressing your feet and your lower back on the mat.

2 Bring your knees up, one at a time to start with on two breaths and then both at once, when this feels right, on one in breath. On your next exhalation, hold your baby on your bent legs. If you are both happy, this is an ideal posture to tone your pelvic floor in depth, drawing in as you inhale and more as you exhale, releasing your muscles only at the end of the exhalation. Repeat six times, if your baby allows. Your baby's weight makes this exercise easier and more effective.

3 Still holding your baby, take a deep breath and come up to a sitting position, pulling your back straight as you exhale. End here or let yourself go back again for another lift in a see-saw rhythm. Again, your baby's weight is a help. Avoid this last practice for three months if you have had a Cesarean section and do not repeat lifts more than three times in one session.

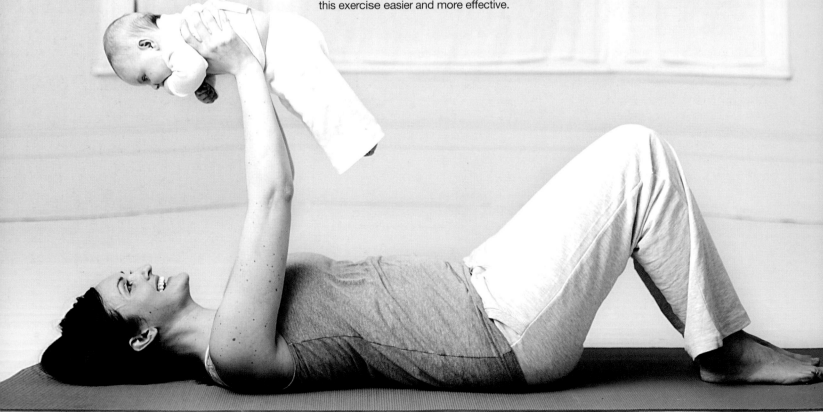

Boat pose

This classic yoga pose is an intense toner of your back and stomach muscles. It is highly energizing. Previous experience of yoga is required to execute the pose fully, but even then do not attempt it until your fourth postnatal month. If you are new to yoga, the first step in the progression below is very beneficial, and the swan pose, shown in Step 4, is a wonderfully relaxing posture that your baby may find intriguing.

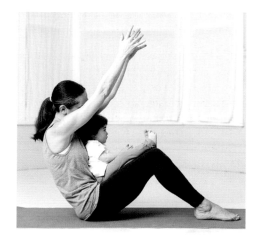

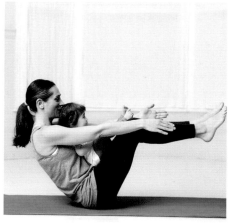

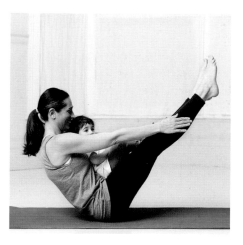

1 Sit on your mat with bent knees together. Sit your baby with her back against your body and her legs extended along your thighs. Stretch your arms out in front of you and breathe deeply in and out—the deeper you breathe, the more you are able to align your spine. This is far more strenuous than it looks. Release your arms and keep breathing deeply.

2 Once you can straighten your back with your feet on the mat, try the next step. Inhale and lift your arms up. As you exhale, lower your arms to extend them horizontally and lift your bent legs to the same level. Your baby is also in boat pose. Hold the pose for a few seconds only, breathing deeply. Come back to a sitting position and release your arms.

3 If you are able to keep your back straight while raising your bent legs, try to straighten them when you lower your arms horizontally on an exhalation. The aim is to stretch your lower back up in a V shape with your extended legs, using deep breathing to hold the pose. Release when you tense up.

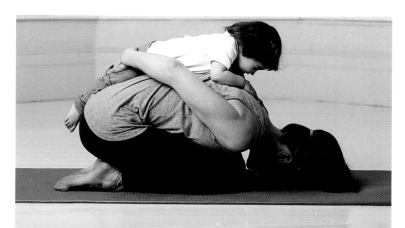

4 Sit on your heels and bend forward with your head on the mat in classic yoga swan pose, a counter to boat pose. If your baby is old enough, hold her on your back to help you stretch. Deep breathing in this pose helps you to relax and to enter a healing space, if this is what you need.

Strengthen your lumbar

Regular practice of this sequence will strengthen your lumbar area, which will inevitably have been weakened, not only by your pregnancy but also by having to carry heavy items of baby equipment. These cat rolls prevent and alleviate back pain. You can turn to them any time your back is getting sore—and seeing you alternately at a distance and close up is very entertaining for your baby. The flowing movement can be regarded as your first grounded sun salutation after giving birth.

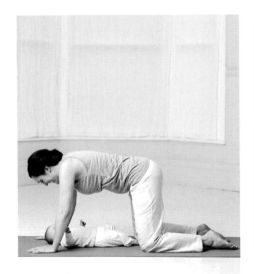 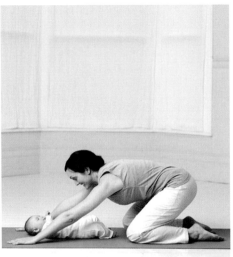 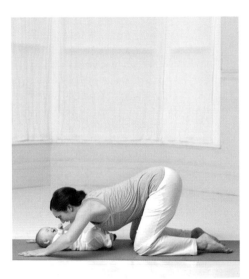

1 Check that your knees are directly under your hips and that your hands are under your shoulders. Your baby is best lying on her back facing you, with her face under yours. Raise your shoulders slightly as you look at your baby to ensure that your back is flat, with your neck and spine in a straight line. This is cat pose.

2 Inhale and as you breathe out lean back, stretching your lower back toward your heels without moving your hands at all.

3 Inhale again and bend your elbows slightly. Use a long exhalation to glide forward with your face hovering over your baby's stomach, chest, and face.

4 Continue stretching forward until your arms are straight. Take a breath to start another round, lifting your shoulders again to roll back.

5 Exhale as you stretch back again toward your heels.

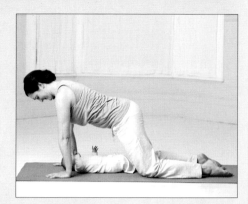 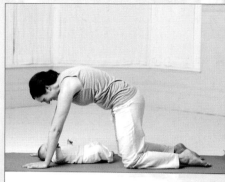

6 Perhaps you can sit on your heels this time before you inhale and glide forward again. Enjoy the feeling of space this creates in your lower back.

Repeat three times and ideally make this a daily morning practice that will be the second cornerstone of your postnatal yoga together with your pelvic-floor toning.

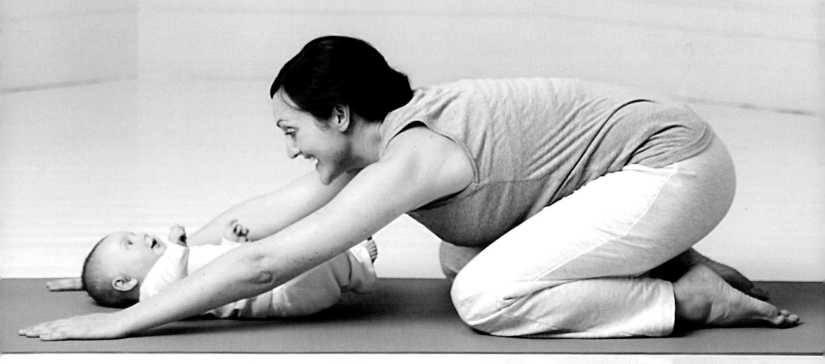

Standing poses

When you feel ready for standing poses, the tall stretch and the classic triangle and forward-stretch poses offer elongations that tone those muscles that you are likely to strain when feeding your baby and carrying her. They will also refresh and energize you in just a few minutes.

Tall stretch

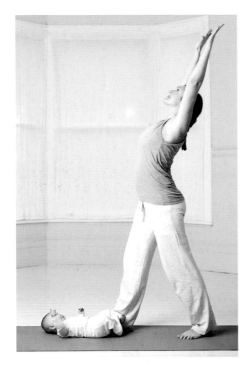 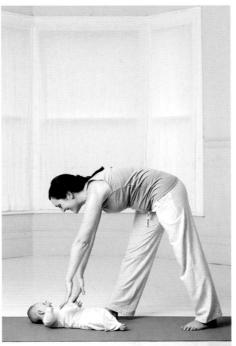 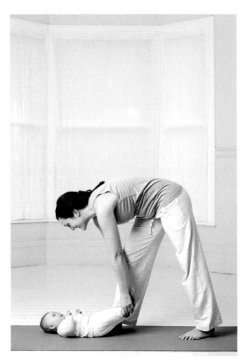

1 With your baby lying on her back in front of you, place one foot next to her feet and step back with your other foot to a comfortable distance. Avoid wide stances because your pelvic ligaments are still soft and vulnerable to overstretching. Inhale and slowly take your arms up in front of you, extending over your head and stretching from feet to finger tips.

2 Exhale as you extend your arms forward and stretch in a wide arch reaching down to your baby while keeping your back foot solidly grounded.

3 Bend your knees if you need to in order to give your baby a long stroke from shoulders to feet. Jiggle her feet lightly to involve her. This stretch can be a single practice if repeated three times.

Easy triangle

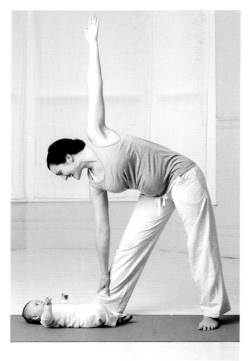

From Step 3 opposite, turn your back foot out, stretch up the arm on the side of your back leg as you inhale, and exhale as you hold the stretch. Place your other hand on your front leg wherever it is comfortable to do so. If possible, turn your head slowly to look up at your hand to get a greater rotation of your chest. Take a breath and lower your arm slowly on your out breath. Jiggle your baby's feet again to say hello and change position to stretch your other side. Then take a short rest in swan pose (page 77) with your baby in front of you.

Simple forward stretch

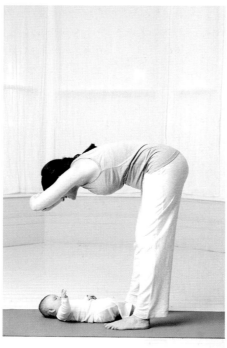

For a relaxed yet effective extension of your whole spine that will complete this short practice, stretch your crossed arms over your head along your ears, holding your elbows. Give your whole back a pleasant stretch while pulling your elbows forward horizontally on each out breath. Make sure that your knees remain soft and bend them slightly if in doubt. Release your arms and say hello to your baby with a nice long stroke.

Classic forward stretch

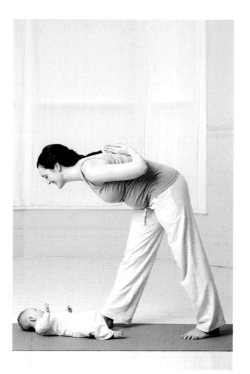

From the basic triangle pose stance, take your hands behind your back, ideally to join palms together against your shoulder blades. Alternatively, hold your elbows behind your back at waist level. Take a breath to stretch forward from your standing position, keeping your back foot solidly grounded. As you exhale, extend horizontally as far as you can above your baby. Stop if you feel that your back curves. Inhale and as you exhale stretch back very slowly to an upright stance. Repeat this stretch with your other leg forward.

Sitting stretches

Re-awaken your whole spine with yoga twists and forward bends that you could not do while you were pregnant. Performed in an upright sitting position, these stretches help release accumulated tension in your shoulders. Sit on a foam block or a phone book to ease your lower back if necessary. Your baby, either sitting against you or lying down facing you, will be a relaxed observer, and gradually copy what you do.

Shoulder stretches

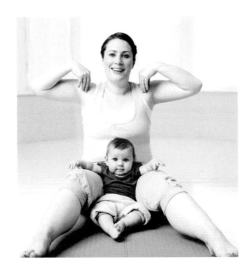

Adjust your sitting position so that your back is as straight as possible. Place your fingers on your shoulders. Inhale and lift your elbows sideways, keeping your neck soft. Exhale and drop your elbows. Feel the weight drop from your shoulders as you repeat this three times.

Shoulder circles

In the same position, circle your elbows, first backward to make space in your chest and then forward to free your upper back. Use the rhythm of your breath to time your movements, lifting on an inhalation and circling on an exhalation.

Open and shut

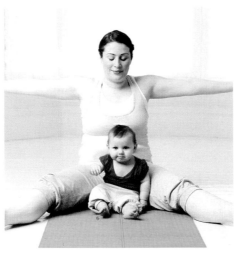

Extend your arms fully in front of you, palms together. Inhale and as you exhale open your arms wide, reaching back as far as you can and stretching out your fingers. Inhale as you return to the starting position. Repeat three times. If you are new to yoga, stretching slowly with the breath may be unfamiliar. Your awareness of reaching deeper muscles grows with practice, and the calm energy that is generated may surprise you.

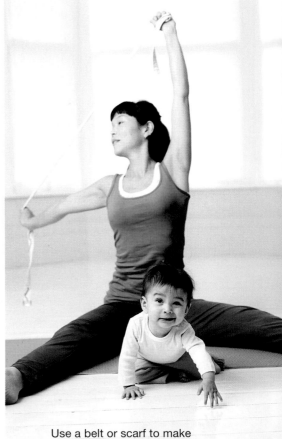

Use a belt or scarf to make this stretch more dynamic, in combination with sideways and circular movements.

Easy forward bend

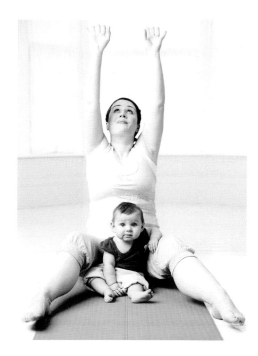

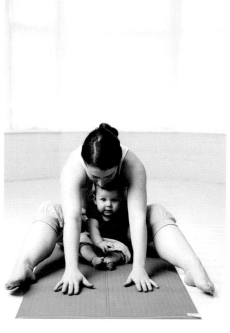

1 From your open stretch, inhale, lift your arms and stretch them over your head, palms facing forward. Look up for further extension as you exhale.

2 Take a breath and as you exhale stretch forward slowly with your arms extended, until your hands reach the mat. Inhale and exhale fully, then release and come up. At first you may need to bend your knees to do this stretch comfortably while stretching your back all the way forward.

Gentle twist

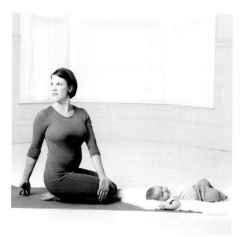

Yoga twists involve a spinal rotation that tones the abdominal and back muscles with the use of the breath, while making space in the upper body. This one helps to bring together parted abdominal muscles (where you feel a gap with your fingers above your navel) and acts on connective tissues in the pelvis. Sit on your heels and place the back of one hand against the outside of your opposite knee. Inhale and take your other arm back to the floor behind you. Using both hands as levers, progressively increase your twist from your lower spine upward with each exhalation. Let your spine lead your head without forcing. You are experiencing yoga's "movement in stillness," which has many known benefits.

Forward bend rowing boat

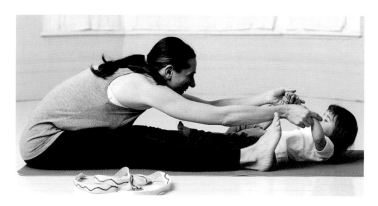

Once your baby can lift herself easily from a lying position, try this playful forward bend, rowing the boat with your baby facing you. Breathe through the rowing movement or sing the rhyme: "Row, row, row your boat gently down the stream, merrily, merrily, merrily, merrily, life is but a dream." Make this stretch easier or more demanding by adjusting the width between your feet. Closing the gap brings you closer to the classic yoga forward bend with an array of beneficial effects, including the slimming of your waist.

Kneeling stretches

These stretches give you a stable base for realigning the curvature of your spine after pregnancy and so help you to recover your poise and balance. Practice slowly at first to derive most benefit from extending your breathing in each stretch, before progressing to a more dynamic rhythm that your baby may find stimulating to follow. Some poses are also beneficial during pregnancy.

Diagonal stretch on all fours

Leg extension and forward bend on all fours

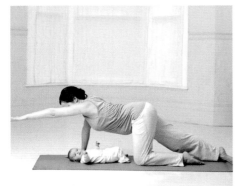 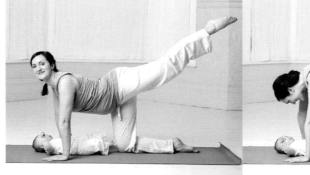 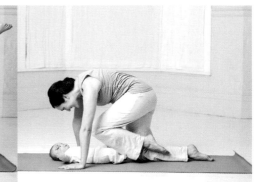

From a stable and aligned cat pose (page 78), inhale and extend one leg back and the opposite arm forward horizontally. Expand this diagonal stretch as you exhale, taking care to keep your hips steady and in line with your knee on the mat. Return to cat pose and loosen your hips to relax your lower back. Repeat three times, following the rhythm of your breath.

1 Make sure that your hands are exactly under your shoulders in cat pose. Breathe in and stretch one leg behind you, horizontally or higher. Exhale into this stretch, keeping your leg relaxed. Either turn your back foot out or extend it, according to how comfortable either stretch feels on your lower back.

2 Breathe in and bring your extended leg forward toward your face, rounding your back. Exhale fully and return to cat pose. Do the same with the other leg and repeat three times. Practice this stretch several times a day if you feel you are developing back pain.

Open wide stretch on all fours

From a stable cat pose, extend one leg back on the mat while turning your hip out. Turn your other knee in and your foot out on the mat to gain stability. Take a breath and extend your arm on the side of your extended leg over your head. This pose is equally beneficial during pregnancy and postnatally, and helps you to expand your breathing and to feel lighter and energized.

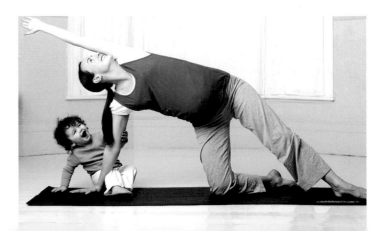

Adapted standing poses

Safe holding is the prerequisite for involving your baby in any standing poses. Take your time at first to shift your baby from one side to the other. Cuddles while you change position are always welcome, and reassurance that he is integral to these poses. As you gain stability, your baby also learns balance.

Eagle pose	High leg bend	Tree pose	Triangle

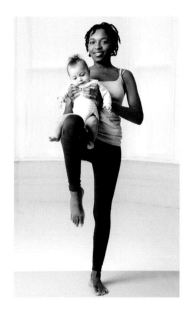 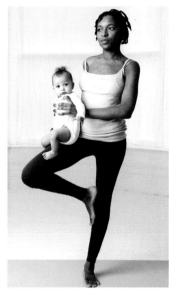 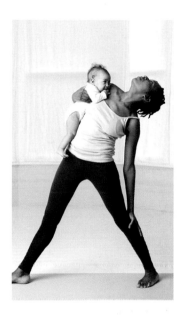

This encourages you to pull in your abdominal muscles as you breathe deeply. With your baby in a cradle hold (page 18), bend your knees and wrap one leg around the other. If you can, tuck your foot behind your calf. Take a full slow breath, focusing on lengthening your exhalation. Undo your legs, take a few relaxing small steps and repeat on the other side.

Hold your baby astride one of your thighs as you raise your knee as high as you can. Keep the foot of your standing leg firmly grounded for a better stretch of your lower back while your upper body remains neutral. A slow practice, with long exhalations, can be very calming, but you can also release tension by turning this pose into an active prancing with a faster breathing rhythm, sliding your baby across as you change legs.

Bring one foot to rest on the inner side of the other leg. Rest your baby high on your thigh, against your body, and take your bent knee right out to the side. If you feel unstable, don't try to hold the pose, and relax with a few small steps as you change sides.

With your baby in shoulder hold, stand with your feet apart, the back one turned in slightly and solidly grounded and your front leg extended. Slide your baby down your side, and when you feel secure holding him against you with one arm, extend your other arm along your back leg. Your baby is helping to stretch your side from hip to shoulder even though your arm is not free to stretch up. Exhale as you return to upright. Relax your legs before repeating the pose on the other side.

Backbend progression

Backbends stretch the front of the body intensely but mostly they stimulate and balance the nervous and endocrine systems. A slow progression from gentle bridge pose to upper backbend is necessary following birth, even if you have years of experience.

Gentle bridge pose

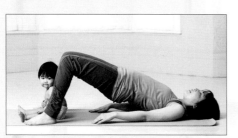

The focus is on your lower back. Take up the bridge pose you use to tone your pelvic floor (page 75). Your baby can sit between your feet. To make the pose more effective, press your hands on the mat on each side of your body. Try to hold the pose for a few cycles of slow breathing, extending your tailbone toward your feet after each round. Repeat three times, then bring your bent knees to your chest and relax your lower back for a moment as a counterpose.

Upper backbend

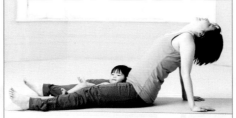

Sit up straight, with your legs slightly apart and your baby between them, resting against you. Put your palms down on the floor behind you and push to stretch your upper back and chest. Breathe deeply. Allowing your head to fall back helps to increase the back stretch, but do this only if it feels comfortable.

Full back stretch

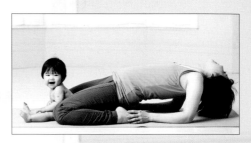

This classic yoga pose can be surprisingly relaxing but it requires suppleness and experience of back stretches. Sit between your heels, your baby between your knees, and gradually lower yourself back to rest on your elbows. Practice this for a couple of weeks, and then reach for your feet and lower your head onto the mat. Breathe deeply for a few cycles and then rest in forward bend (page 77), being careful to avoid putting pressure on your back as you change position.

Caution

Backbends are not advisable during pregnancy and you need to prepare both your lower and upper back before starting them postnatally. Don't attempt a full backbend for at least six months after giving birth.

Relax

Relaxation is an essential component of any yoga practice, when the benefits of the poses are consolidated. Relax in swan (page 77) or corpse pose, especially after a full back stretch.

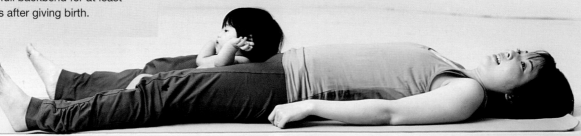

5 Baby Yoga for Enhancing Mobility

In the first eighteen months after birth, all babies have to find their own way of rolling, sitting, and moving around. Some develop crawling skills, some do not, before learning how to stand and finally discovering that they can walk. Each culture supports its babies differently during this time. Cross-cultural studies have shown that babies in less economically advantaged parts of the world can score just as well as, or even better than, affluent babies if they receive appropriate physical stimulation from loving carers. Being held, massaged, and played with on a bare earth floor may actually work better than all our contraptions and developmental toys. Baby yoga helps us to be alert to our babies' triumphs when they have breakthroughs with their body control, and their frustrations when they do not. Once your baby spends time holding her feet and taking them to her mouth, for instance, she is ready to discover new ways of rolling sideways. We are our babies' favorite witnesses. They bask in our appreciation not just of their new achievements but of their own delight. In this chapter, specific resources are presented to help you catch these magical moments. Perhaps they will also help you assist your baby in bringing them about.

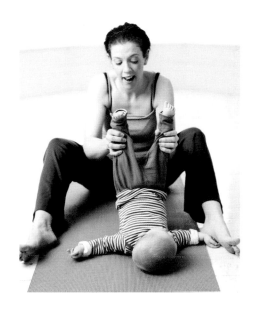

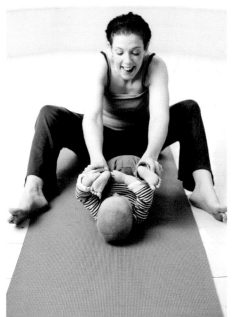

Active hip sequence

This combines familiar moves in a playful sequence of stretches, to help your premobile baby enjoy his energy and cope with his frustrations. If you start yoga with your baby at this stage, go to the dynamic hip sequence (pages 54–55) first, and integrate each of the active hip sequence movements one by one. If your baby refuses to be on his back, you can adapt the dynamic hip sequence to a sitting position.

1 Plow pose

In this pose, your baby's legs are extended toward the floor behind his head, which will help him to develop his lower back muscles. The pose also activates your baby's thyroid gland and helps with digestion, circulation, and respiration. Babies with a tendency to constipation may become more mobile with regular practice of the plow, but avoid it after a feed. When your baby raises his legs while lying on his back, hold them above the knees to help him extend them, without ever forcing. Keep his tailbone on the mat with a very gentle pressure in order to elongate his spine, then release. If he is happy, extend his legs above his face (see photographs on page 87.)

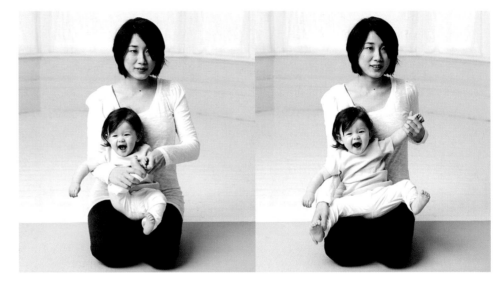

2 Foot tapping

Rather than gently bringing your baby's hand toward his opposite foot, aim at a vigorous diagonal stretch repeated rhythmically. Your baby cannot do this himself, but he will love you helping him.

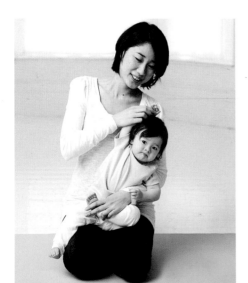

3 Half-lotus stretch

This stretches your baby's side from his extended foot to his hand above his head, introducing him to movements that he cannot yet coordinate but is already attempting. Try to create a steady rhythm as you change sides, and respect your baby's resistance, particularly in the upward arm stretch.

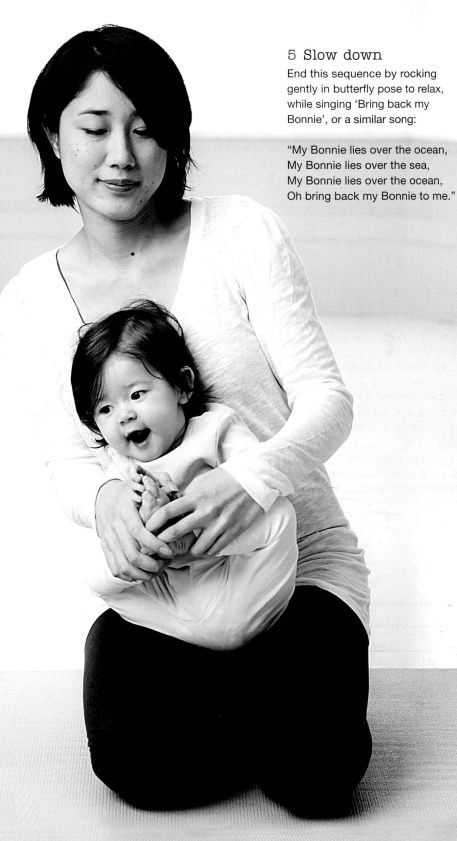

5 Slow down

End this sequence by rocking gently in butterfly pose to relax, while singing 'Bring back my Bonnie', or a similar song:

"My Bonnie lies over the ocean,
My Bonnie lies over the sea,
My Bonnie lies over the ocean,
Oh bring back my Bonnie to me."

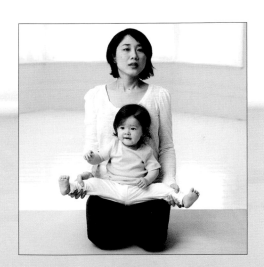

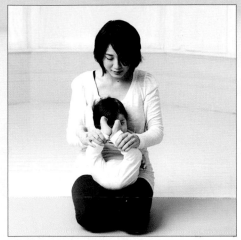

4 Up to the nose

Sit your baby high up on your lap, with his back closely against you, to prevent him slipping. Alternately open your baby's legs wide and bring them together, up to his nose. You can also cross your baby's legs over each other (twice) as part of this movement.

Consolidating your baby's sitting

Be led by your baby in helping him to secure his sitting with enjoyable games. There is no rush, he will sit when he is ready. Whether he does this sooner or later does not reflect his intelligence, just his individuality. He may then go on to try kneeling, stretching forward, and maybe crawling.

Back support in butterfly pose

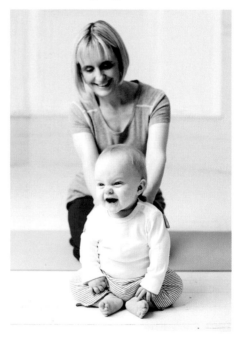

Gently but firmly supporting your baby's lower back with your flat hands will offer him a helpful resistance to strengthen his lower back and develop a stable sitting base.

Arm swings

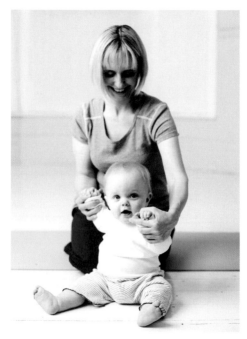

Swing your baby's arms rhythmically, gently at first and then in a more dynamic way, to help stabilize his sitting through a fun movement. One rhyme you could use is:

"Hi Ho, Hi Ho, it's off to work we go
Hi Ho, Hi Ho, Hi Ho."

Hand taps

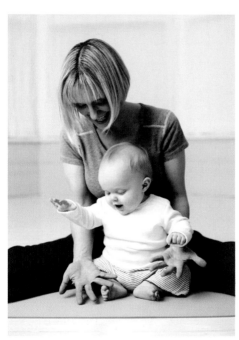

All babies love hand games. Whether your baby needs you to guide his hand or is able to do it himself, clapping games help him to enjoy the transition between supported sitting and unaided sitting.

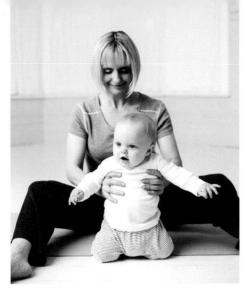

Shoulder hold

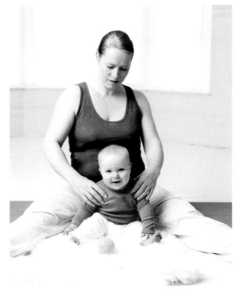

Once your baby starts sitting unaided for short moments, the gentle pressure of your hands on her shoulders helps her to open her chest and move her spine more freely in a sitting position. This will create lifelong foundations for a strong posture, with all the associated health benefits.

Mini hero pose

Many babies like to kneel-sit between their feet in a mini version of the classic hero pose. Holding your baby firmly under the arms, help him to raise himself up and then release so that he sits back between his feet. Repeat a few times if this is something your baby is trying to achieve, because it will help him in his attempts to crawl later on.

Paddle to the ball

A lot of babies show us how they progress from sitting to crawling, via kneeling, if we watch. It is common to see babies sitting with one leg extended forward and one leg bent backward, particularly if they are eager to reach a goal. Diagonal paddling arm stretches help your sitting baby to gain more strength and impetus to extend her own arm and launch forward to discover crawling. She will soon find her way to the ball…

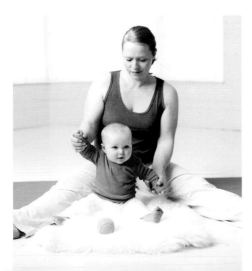

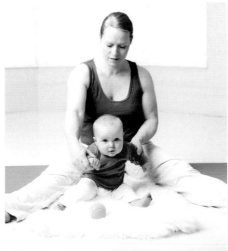

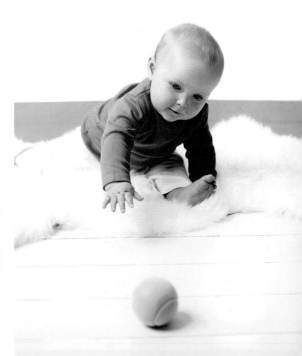

Help your baby to crawl

These holds help your baby to keep the whole front of her body relaxed while using her back in her attempts to crawl. Giving your baby a very slight lift helps her gain an awareness of the completion of moves that she has already nearly mastered.

Ribcage lift

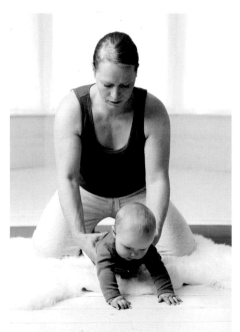

Once your baby can reach forward to the floor while sitting in butterfly or kneeling in hero pose, place your hands on the sides of her ribcage with your fingers supporting her chest and your thumbs extended just under her shoulder blades. Alternately apply gentle pressure with your thumbs and your fingers, resulting in a small lift of her whole upper body while her hands remain on the mat.

Shoulder lift

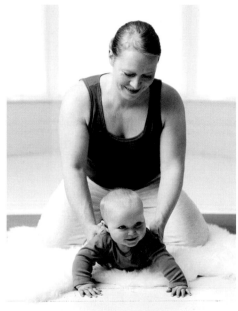

Modify the previous hold by bringing your thumbs slightly lower under your baby's shoulder blades. This helps her to lift her upper body and push off from her hands, as in the classic cobra pose, and eases the forward extension of her arms. She is now lying on her stomach as her legs have extended back from her initial all-fours position.

Shoulder take off

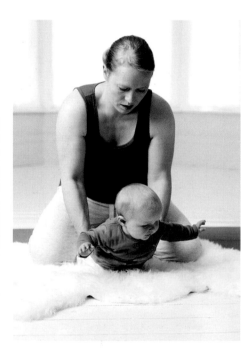

Move your hands still lower on your baby's back. The pressure helps her to lift her arms and her upper body from the floor if she is ready. Slide your hands under her arms to support her, without lifting her any further than she is able to lift herself. Allow her to release when she has had enough.

Hip support

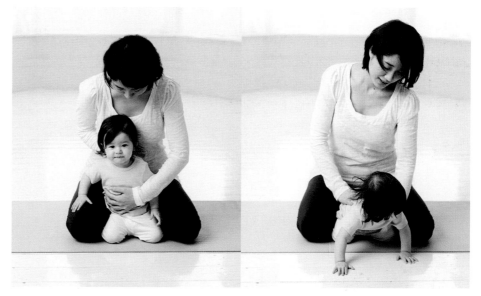

If your baby extends forward freely from kneeling but then is static and gets frustrated, slide one of your hands under her hips for a slight support. This is often enough to release movement from her lower spine. Do not lift her hips because this might make her tip forward.

Hero gets going

Supporting your baby's stomach and back may give him just the resistance he needs to take off after gathering strength in long bouts of hero kneeling over the previous weeks. Enjoy both his and your surprise at this newfound freedom.

Scooping start

Sometimes babies keep falling back on their front in their attempts at crawling. If this is what your baby does, kneel beside her and slide one hand under her chest and one under her hips. Inhale and lift her lightly, allowing her to keep her hands and feet on the floor. Do not take her weight. This may help to free her leg movements for crawling.

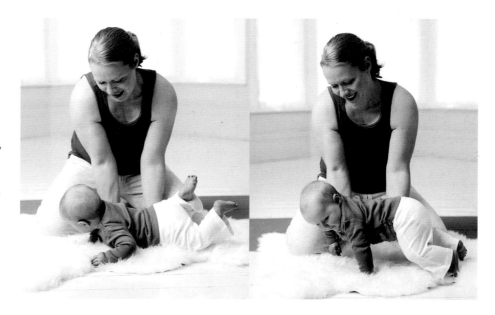

Further encouragement

It sometimes seems to take a long time for babies to move on from the nearly crawling stage to full mobility. There is no hurry. Your baby has to integrate a whole range of versatile movements into the purposeful action of crawling, and each baby does this slightly differently. Not all babies crawl—some go straight to standing. There are, however, benefits to crawling and it is probably better to have this experience. The baby yoga stretches presented here help babies who are nearly there.

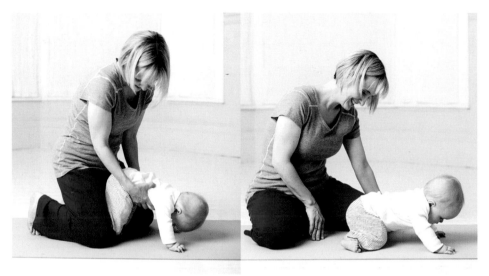

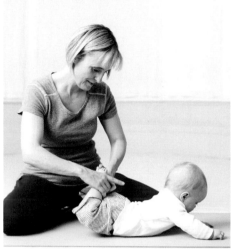

If, from a kneeling start, your baby extends his arms forward and moves only slightly, try lifting his hips to free his leg movement.

If your baby still needs help to move his legs under his body, gently extend and lift his legs, holding his feet together over his buttocks. This enhances his back strength and flexibility.

Also, extend one leg back at a time …

… and then take the knee forward, holding your baby's lower leg while stabilizing his hip with your other hand. This may be all he needs to use his legs efficiently in a forward—or, at first, backward—crawling movement.

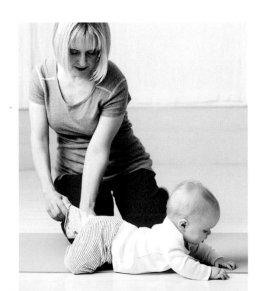

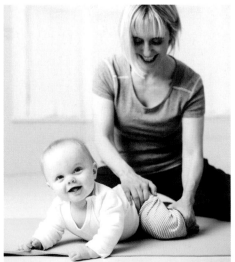

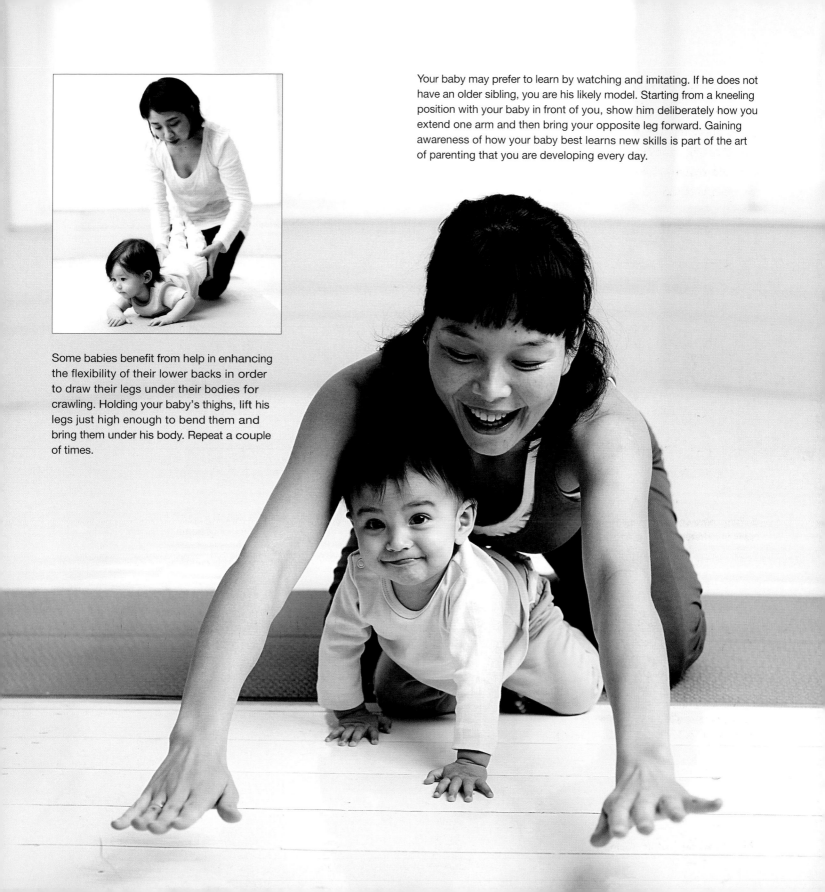

Your baby may prefer to learn by watching and imitating. If he does not have an older sibling, you are his likely model. Starting from a kneeling position with your baby in front of you, show him deliberately how you extend one arm and then bring your opposite leg forward. Gaining awareness of how your baby best learns new skills is part of the art of parenting that you are developing every day.

Some babies benefit from help in enhancing the flexibility of their lower backs in order to draw their legs under their bodies for crawling. Holding your baby's thighs, lift his legs just high enough to bend them and bring them under his body. Repeat a couple of times.

Secure standing

Your baby's attempts to stand may have been less noticeable than his efforts to crawl on his hands and knees, or shuffle around on his bottom, but once he can pull himself up, he will soon be standing. It is important to continue providing effective support to ease his transition to walking, which will reduce considerably the number of his falls and therefore his distress. The principles of yoga guide the following easy, interactive practices. Try them while you are playing with him.

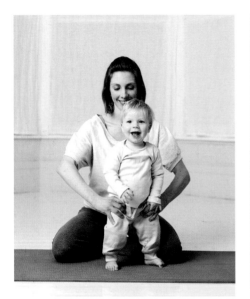

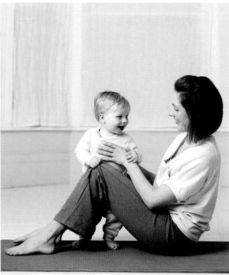

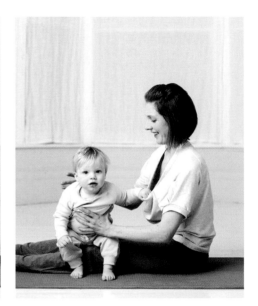

Stand your baby on his feet in front of you, facing out. Place your hands on his hips, extending your fingers inward, and use your thumbs at the back of his hips to exert slight downward pressure. Babies are usually happy with this stabilizing action, at least for a few seconds.

Sit on your mat and stand your baby sideways in front of you between your legs. Bring your knees up and use them to hold him upright. Rest your hands on his chest and upper back to complement the support of your knees.

Sit on the mat with your legs straight out in front of you, and sit your baby on one of your thighs, facing out. A gentle backward dip will encourage him to spring up to his feet while you support him with your hands on his chest and upper back. Repeat a couple of times.

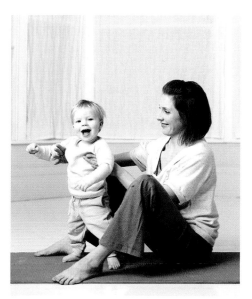

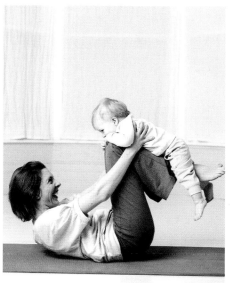

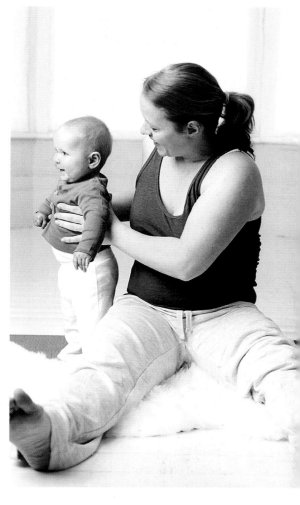

Raise your knees in a sitting position. Perch your baby on the front edge of one of them and let him slide down your leg to plant his feet on the ground. To lift your baby without strain, sit him on your knee while your leg is straight and inhale as you raise it. Avoid this practice if you are pregnant.

Your baby may be familiar with baby flier (page 76). Now you can use this practice as a standing balance. Sitting with your knees up, place your baby upright against your legs, facing you. Hold him under the arms, roll back, and use your momentum to sit back up again. Your baby can use his feet to push from the floor as you roll back and up again. If you are energetic, this can become a see-saw movement that your baby will find exhilarating besides helping him to stand.

If your baby is not too heavy, you can help her to stand as part of your yoga sitting practice. If she stands up easily from sitting on one of your thighs, hold her sides firmly and lift her across your legs like a rainbow to land on the outside of your other thigh. Loosen your hold to help her find her stance. She may wobble or sit down. After a few lifts your baby may enjoy squatting in anticipation of her next rainbow crossing.

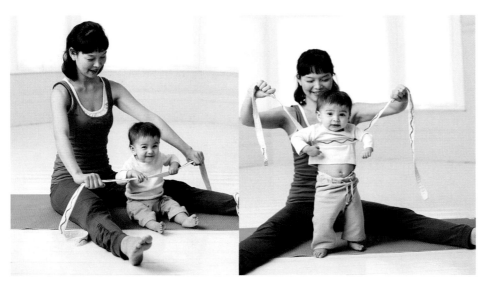

If you like stretching with a belt, you can use it to help him practice his standing. With your baby sitting in front of you, have him take hold of the belt. If he already stands unaided, lifting the belt will help him stretch up to standing. If he cannot yet do this, slide the belt under his arms to give him a lift. Once he stands, relax your hold and let your baby find his stance.

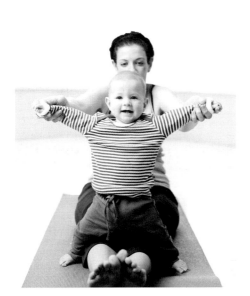

Sit on your mat and stand your baby in front of you. Put one of your legs between his legs and give him a little lift off the floor, then lower his feet onto the mat, supporting him under his arms against your raised knee. Your baby may want a repeat. The lower toward your ankle he sits on your leg, the more strenuous for you. Avoid this practice if you are newly pregnant.

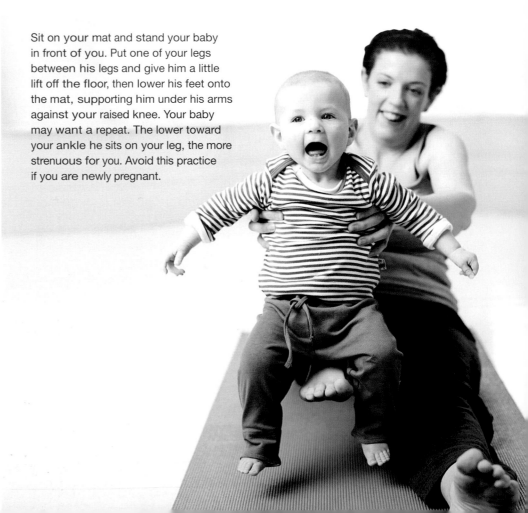

Sit with your legs extended in front of you and bend your knees slightly so that your baby can sit on your legs, just below your knees, with his feet on the mat on each side of you. Hold his hands. Inhale, drop your knees and stretch out your baby's arms so that he stands in an X shape. Exhale and loosen your arms. He may sit back and want more. Make this practice dramatic and exciting!

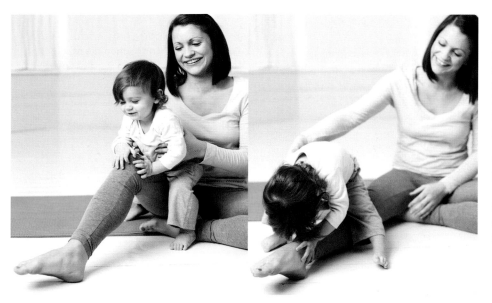

Many babies like "horsie" rides. If you sit on the floor and have your baby ride across one of your legs, these games can help him root his feet solidly and gain better balance. Bend your leg so that you can use your foot to create movement without strain. Try the popular rhyme:

"Horsie horsie don't you stop
Let your feet go clippety clop"

Surprise your baby now and again with a drop of your knee and help him regain his balance with a laugh.

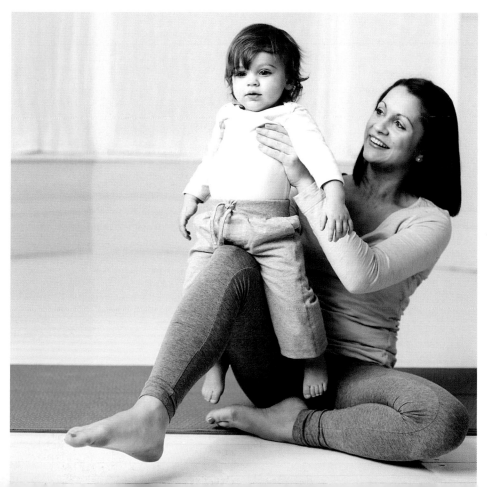

Sit your baby on one of your knees, holding him under the arms. Take a breath and raise your knee so that his feet come off the ground. Exhale and bring your foot back to the floor so that he lands solidly on his feet. He will find the combination of a balance and then grounding enjoyable.

Dynamic inversions for nearly mobile babies

Once babies start standing, they often enjoy a wider range of movement that in turn helps them to gain greater flexibility and strength in their preparation for walking. Tumbles are among babies' favorite games at this stage, and you can take pride in your yoga baby's down dog pose as he goes head down for sheer pleasure.

Dynamic inversions in which your baby lands on his feet allow him to find his centering again, good experience for the rougher tumbles that he will inevitably get into later on. Be guided by your baby's enjoyment of this new experience, and repeat a dynamic inversion no more than twice at a time—and then enjoy a cuddle.

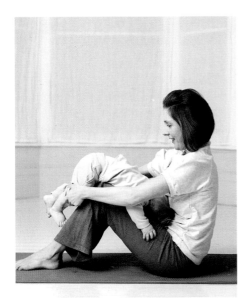 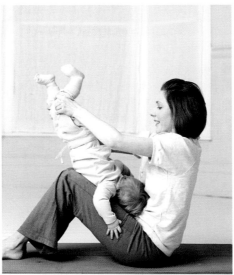 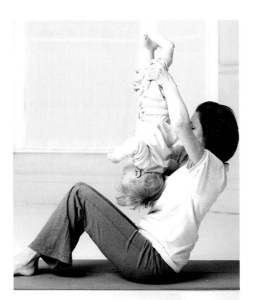

1 Sit on your mat and stand your baby between your knees, holding him under the arms. Bring your knees up under his hips so that he balances on your bent legs in an inverted V shape with his head close to your stomach.

2 Take a firm hold of your baby's legs with both your hands and lift them up to a vertical position.

3 In one continuous movement, take a deep breath and lift your baby up from your lap, leaning back slightly to make this lift easier for you.

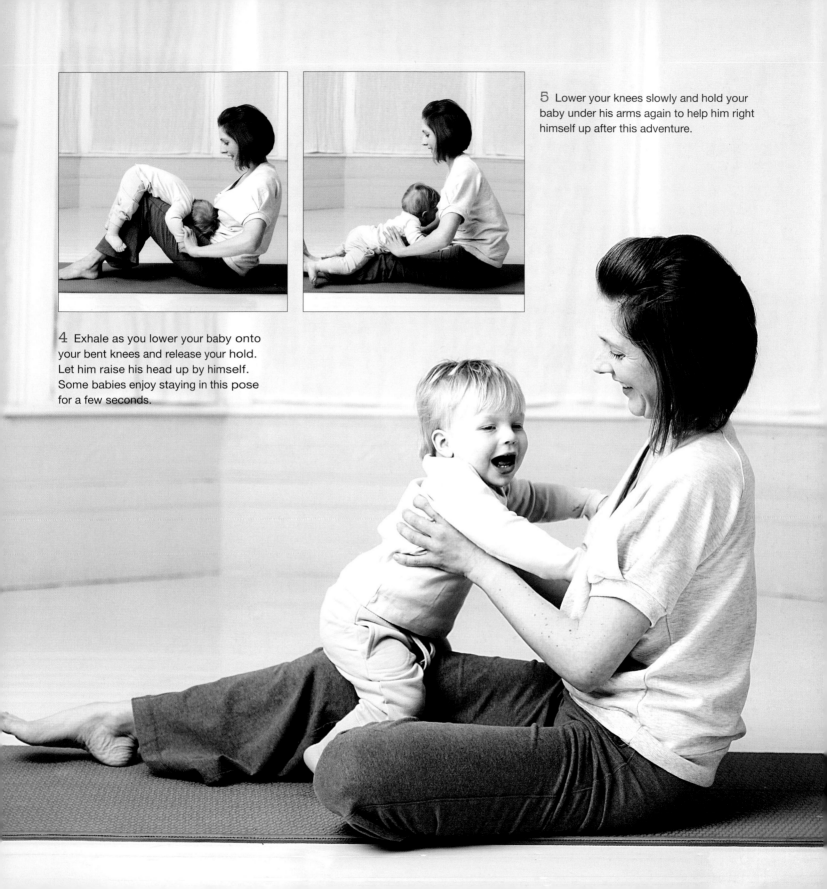

5 Lower your knees slowly and hold your baby under his arms again to help him right himself up after this adventure.

4 Exhale as you lower your baby onto your bent knees and release your hold. Let him raise his head up by himself. Some babies enjoy staying in this pose for a few seconds.

Special babies

Alignment is the key for babies with special needs. Straightening your baby's spine as much as possible, to where is naturally comfortable for her, and making sure her hips are as level and her head as straight as possible means her body will be starting in the most supported position. Use a rolled towel under one side of her body if necessary to level her hips. Children with Down's syndrome, cerebral palsy, or related conditions may have instability in their hips, so avoid any postures that can overextend this area. For babies with severe reflux during a massage or hip sequence, use a rolled towel under the head and upper body, to make lying down more comfortable.

For babies who have a gastrostomy tube or peg, "tummy time" is still important, as are exercises that include holds or rolling where pressure will be placed on this area. Be extra careful, especially if surgery is recent or there is an infection making the area sore, and always watch her cues closely. Some babies may seem to have limited means of communication but they are clear in relaying their need to stop. Check the gestures on page 14. These are your baby's cues. Refer to them frequently but note that for babies with cerebral palsy, turning the head away and alternately flexing and extending the legs is normal, so look for other cues.

Caution

Adult-led inversions should be avoided if your baby has:
- Epilepsy or non-diagnosed fitting, including minor absences.
- Cardiac problems, depending on severity.
- Any skeletally unstable condition, including hip instability.
- A ventricular shunt—a tube that drains excess cerebrospinal fluid from the brain to relieve excess pressure.

If your baby has heart irregularities, be careful with inversions and slow down moving exercises to avoid overstimulation.

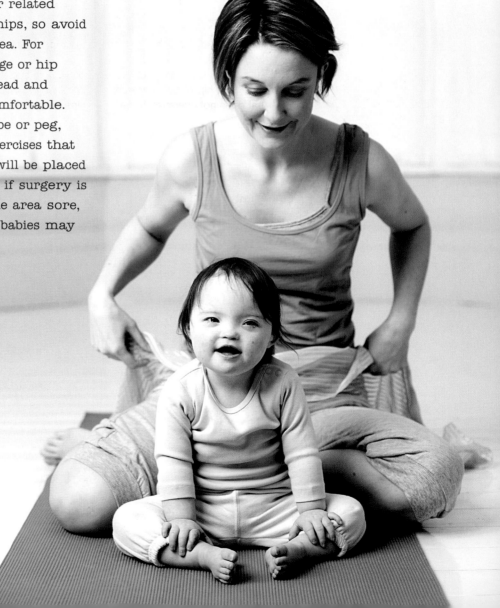

Helpful exercises

Sitting your baby in an aligned position helps to strengthen the muscles around hips and legs. A baby with Down's syndrome will often sit naturally with legs bent outward. Those with cerebral palsy related conditions may adopt a similar pose but usually with more limb stiffness, or both legs may roll over to one side.

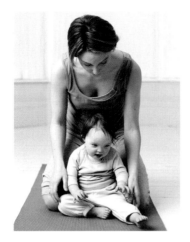

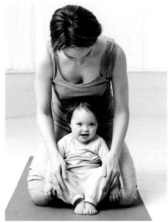

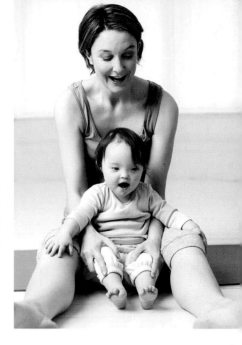

Bending one leg out at a time is a gentle hip-opening exercise that does not overstretch the joints. If the bent leg is stiff, use a rolled towel under the thigh and knee to offer support. Encourage your baby to lean forward and touch her toes, or to reach as far as is comfortable. Practice this on each side, not just the stiff side.

Sit your baby between your knees so you can support her hips as much as necessary. This position is good for encouraging her to flatten her feet on the yoga mat.

With your baby sitting between your knees, peddle one of her legs at a time toward her chest —perhaps incorporate a song or chant. You could do this with your baby lying down but supported sitting works the muscles much more deeply, and is best for a baby with severe reflux. It is also a good position for you to practice slow, gentle breathing together.

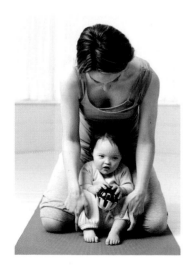

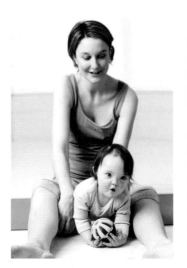

One way to encourage an aligned position, and hand-eye coordination, is to sit opposite a mirror (or another parent and baby) and encourage your baby to roll out and reach for a ball.

If your baby cannot sit unsupported, place your open hands around her hips while she sits in butterfly pose, with the soles of her feet together. This may not be appropriate for a baby who has hip instability, but be guided by your child and pay attention (as always) to her cues. If she shows any discomfort at all, stop and gently put her in a more comfortable aligned position, as above.

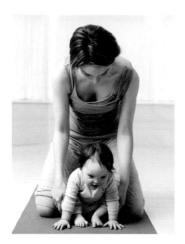 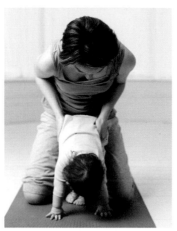 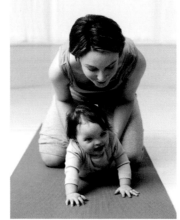 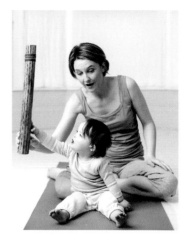

If your baby is able to do inversions (see box, page 102), dog pose can help increase flexibility without overstretching. The feet should be flat on the floor but some babies may find this challenging, especially those with cerebral palsy because they can suffer with shortening of the tendons. Help your baby into the pose by lifting and holding her hips. If dog pose is not possible, alternate flexion and pointing of the feet helps to lengthen and strengthen a weakened or stiff ankle joint and so to encourage walking.

Cobra pose not only opens the chest, and gives the back a beautiful stretch, it also encourages head control and works the shoulders, arms, and hands. It is especially good for a baby with cerebral palsy, because it encourages alignment and can really help stiff hands to open up against gentle pressure on the yoga mat. Support your baby's hips with your thighs to enable her to lift her upper body as much as she can.

Children with cerebral palsy often have a one-sided weakness, so it is important to encourage them to use both sides. An Amazonian rainmaker stick (not to be used without supervision) can help, or use a rattle, or just your voice.

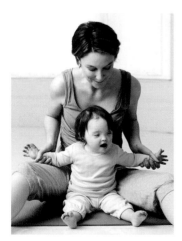 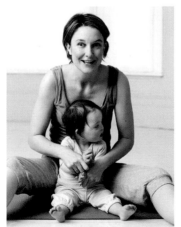

Criss-crossing arms gives a lovely stretch and also helps with coordination. If your baby's shoulders are stiff, try with one arm at a time. Place a hand on her shoulder for support as you open and close each arm. Don't open her arm or cross over farther than she can comfortably go.

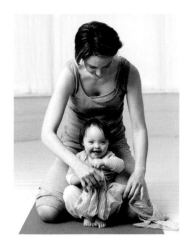

Peeping games are good for hand-eye coordination, and an opaque scarf is a useful prop. Put it on your baby's head and wait for her to remove it. If she finds this difficult, help her by putting your hand over hers, but encourage her to pull the scarf away herself. Sit her in an aligned position if possible, with her legs bent or straight out in front.

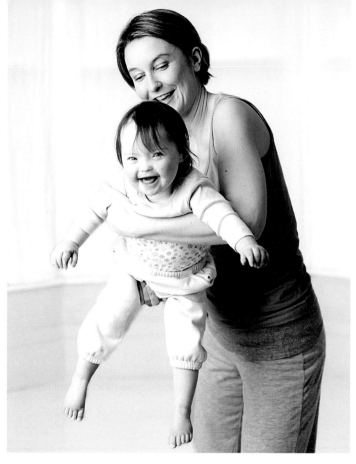

A supported swing puts less pressure on the hips, and on the abdomen for those babies with severe reflux or a new gastrostomy tube or peg.

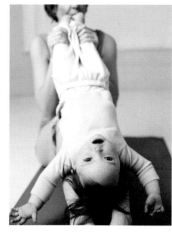

A supported inversion (see box, page 102) is best done sitting on the floor. Lie your baby along your legs and, holding her ankles, or around her torso if she is wriggly, gently bend your knees until she is lying down your shins. This stretches her spine safely. Encouraging her to relax and release her arms opens her chest—especially good for children who have a closed and stiff posture. You could hold your baby around the hips, but not if she has hip instability.

Breathing for relaxation

Sit comfortably, either in a chair or on the floor, leaning against a wall. Put your baby on your knee, with her back to your stomach. Hug her around her middle and notice her breathing. Inhale, pause, and then breathe out. See if you can synchronize your breathing and notice how relaxing this becomes. Close your eyes if you wish but keep your focus—the point is not to fall asleep! This practice relaxes the breath, the mind, and the body.

Singing or chanting to your baby, and supporting this with a hand sign, encourages focus and prepares you both for relaxation.

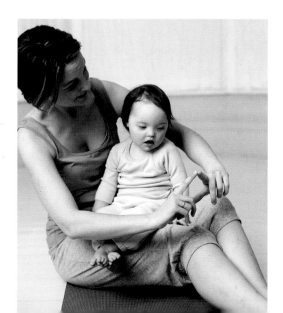

Relax together

This is an essential component of yoga with your nearly mobile baby. He may be constantly on the move, but he is becoming more attuned to contrasts between quiet and activity, rough and gentle, fast and slow, and your self-awareness continues to be central to his development. Even the most indefatigable premobile babies appreciate times of stillness and rest when they take stock. As they grow, babies are increasingly sensitive to changes in your voice, breathing patterns, and rhythms. Developing calm modes of interaction will help you to introduce, or deepen, relaxation time with your baby, and prepare him for sleeping through teething and changing routines. Here are various practical suggestions.

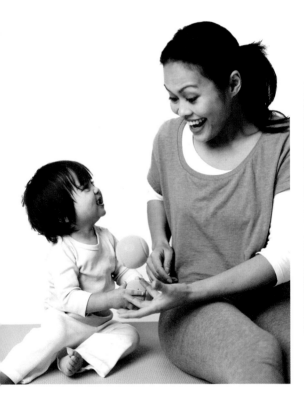

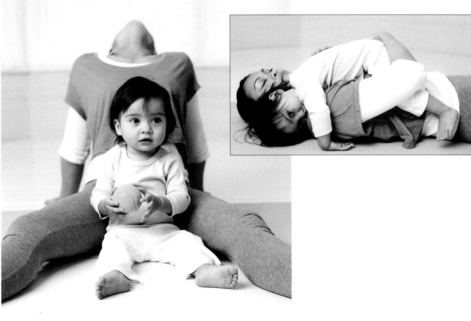

First of all, your baby needs to feel that he has got your total attention. Make a commitment to absolutely necessary interruption only. The quality of your engagement determines your baby's response—the toy is just a support.

Slow down your breathing and focus on the moment. If your baby starts scooting around, fetches other objects, or tries to climb all over you, let him do so. You are already relaxing and he will notice your change of consciousness. One object may then become the center of his attention. Trust that you were truly here with him was needed for him to engage single-mindedly with a toy. Now you can deepen your own relaxation, releasing accumulated tension. Extending your exhalations in a sitting backbend can be instantly refreshing. Drop your head back if this feels comfortable. If your baby is happy, lie down and relax fully.

Hand mudras

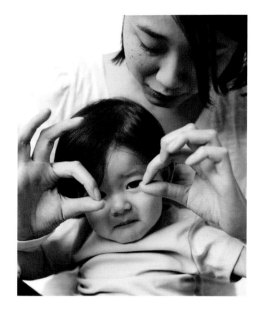

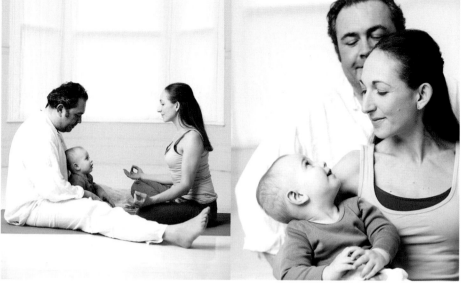

Yoga includes many formalized hand gestures, called mudras, which have been passed down in the Indian tradition because of their reported physiological benefits. Practicing mudras with your baby induces quiet concentration. You may be surprised to see him replicate your mudras unexpectedly weeks later, out of the blue.

From their time in the womb, babies love the combination of their parents' voices. Try yoga chanting as a family. A simple phrase in celebration of the lotus flower, padmi, can get you started: "O-O-Om Om Padmi Om."

Find your own way to chant this phrase, repeating it many times in different keys and changing your pitch. If you enjoy this practice, buy a CD of chants. Humming familiar tunes that you find soothing can also signal relaxation time to your baby.

Drawing inward

This classic yoga practice is easy to learn and can help you relax deeply while still remaining attentive to what your baby is doing. First, give out clear signals to your baby that this is relaxation time—a box of small soft toys that you produce specifically at this time and then put away with your yoga mat can keep him occupied as you relax. At the same time, he will be watching you and deciding between being close to you and exploring. If your baby is a tentative sitter, back him up with a couple of cushions. He may try to move away and need help, so be prepared to be interrupted at any time.

1 Start by closing your eyes for a few seconds, relying on your hearing to sense your baby. Open them briefly for a check and then close them again. Repeat this a few times, gradually keeping your eyes closed for longer. Your baby may register that you are entering a sleep-like state.

2 The next step is to draw your hearing inward. With your eyes closed, be aware of all the sounds around you, particularly any sound that your baby may be producing. Focus on a regular sound in the background—a ticking clock, sounds of nature or of traffic—to heighten your awareness of space and sound together.

3 Soften the palm of your hands to draw in your sense of touch. Register what your baby is doing and if he comes close, hold him loosely without stroking him or talking to him.

4 Finally, relax your lower jaw. Exhale deeply, relax your facial muscles with a soft smile and be aware of your senses of taste and smell. If your baby allows it, continue with a full relaxation. Tips with this practice are not to mind either being interrupted or diverting your full attention from relaxing to caring mode.

6 Mobile Babies

Mobility opens new perspectives for your baby, but he needs your anchorage to feel secure before launching himself off to explore. This is a time of consolidation and integration for both of you. Your baby may welcome a different style of massage and communication with touch. As a playful, interactive practice, baby yoga offers an invaluable foundation for development. Picking him up continues to be a main application of yoga in your day-to-day living—an opportunity to tone your pelvic muscles, strengthen your back, and use your breathing fully. For your baby, being picked up cheerfully instantly opens a new interactive space. Assist his first steps without strain, and watch how he imitates your movements. Your readiness to be receptive and respond to him is crucial. His rhythms are now faster than yours and in each practice he starts to play out the humor and drama implicit in earlier baby yoga sequences. How much fun can you give yourself permission to have? How much are you prepared to learn? Assisting your baby's individual discovery of himself at this pre-verbal stage adds a fertile and positive layer for his future self-esteem and wellbeing in the world.

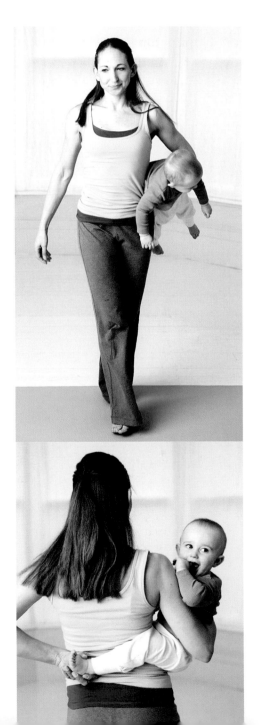

Picking up your baby

Walking with your baby resting on your hip face down (opposite page) may seem undignified but it is extremely comfortable for you both. You can turn this bundle hold into hip stride by rotating him so that he is upright with a leg on either side of your body, sitting on the crest of your hip rather than in the hollow of your waist. To help his positioning and check your spinal alignment, reach out for his back foot with your free hand and straighten yourself now and again (opposite page).

A high lift

As your baby gets heavier, protecting your lower back as you pick him up becomes a priority. The way you pick him up matters to him, too. He feels your weariness or your upbeat energy.

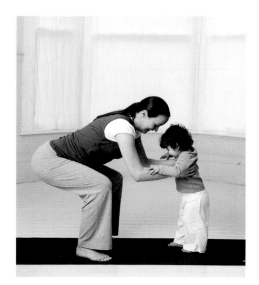 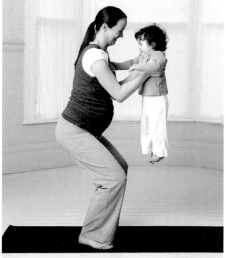 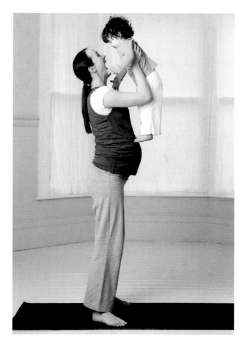

1 The more solidly grounded you are, the lighter your baby will feel. Bend your knees and extend your back into a comfortable semi squat, with your feet parallel on the floor, not much more than hip-width apart. Practice without your baby at first, taking care to align your head with your spine as you extend your arms forward. Inhale, exhale as you stretch back, and inhale again as you come back to an upright position.

2 Speed and momentum are crucial to the fluidity of your up-lift and this is where breathing will help you most. Visualize an uninterrupted scooping movement in which you lift your baby on your way back up. Have your arms bent as you get hold of his sides firmly under his arms and "breathe" him up, keeping your knees bent and your back straight.

3 Continue with a high lift over your head in a full extension of your abdominal and back muscles. This is particularly helpful if your muscles have separated during pregnancy and even more if you are pregnant again, and is exhilarating for your baby.

Reintroducing body massage

As babies set off to discover the world around them, resistance to lying still for a massage is very common. The more you insist on a routine that weeks ago gave you both so much enjoyment, the more wriggling and confrontation you may generate. Through this period, it is more positive to take the chance of a short foot, hand, or head massage as part of a cuddle. The time for full body massage will come again when your baby is ready. Be prepared to change position, strokes, rhythms, and mood to suit his more grown-up needs, although the soothing nursery rhymes of early babyhood often produce instant calming responses.

Sitting long stroke

In order to establish that this is a new style of massage, sit your baby in front of you, facing out. Watch the interest that he is taking in his body and in the sensations of your massage. He may have become ticklish around his stomach or under his feet; his navel may be a new focus of curiosity. Rediscover your baby's body with him in the process of reintroducing massage.

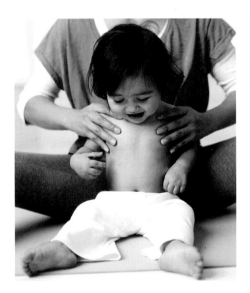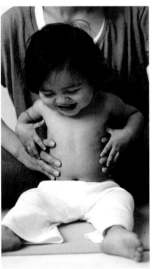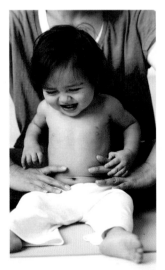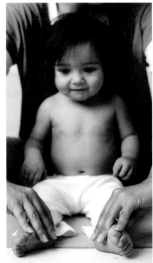

1 Place your hands on his shoulders and gently knead the base of his neck with your thumbs. A relaxed response will indicate receptivity. As ever, it is important to respect a refusal. He may move away, and then come back to sit in front of you, letting you know that this is now done on his terms.

2 Making use of palms and fingers, stroke your baby firmly down the whole front of his body, moving from his upper chest to his feet in one long continuous stroke, exhaling as you do so. Repeat this three times.

Standing back rub

This is a combined squeeze and rub for your baby's back muscles, and may be particularly welcomed by babies affected by coughs and chest congestion. Try it first with dry hands and then, if his response is positive, have your oil ready to signal that this is massage again in a different form.

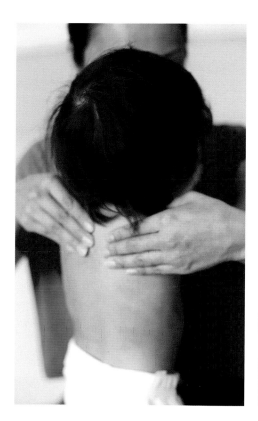 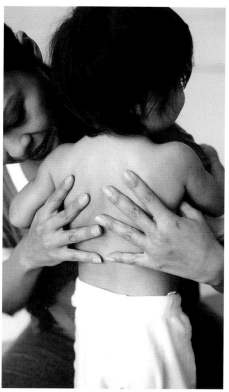 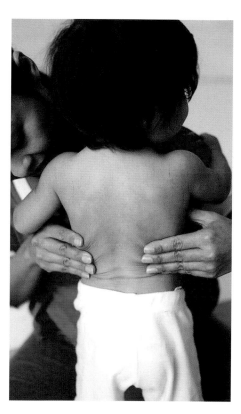

1 Some mobile babies respond better to a deeper kneading of their backs as a way of reintroducing massage. First make contact by placing both of your hands on his shoulders and gently kneading the base of his neck with your fingers.

2 If you get a "go ahead" response, extend your hands on your baby's back, using all the pads of your fingers and keeping your thumbs neutral on his chest.

3 With your fingers together, stroke down his back and then to the side before moving your hands back up to his shoulder blades.

Back massage

Once your baby enjoys the long stroke and back rub, he may be ready for a new massage routine. Let him show you with his body language as he sits or stands relaxed and still, seeking closeness with you. Be careful not to impose it too early, or you may be met with a blunt refusal. Start in a simple and straightforward way. It is easier to have your baby across your legs, as is done traditionally in most parts of the world, although you may wish to use a towel to protect your clothes from oil stains.

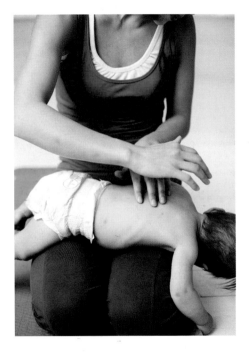 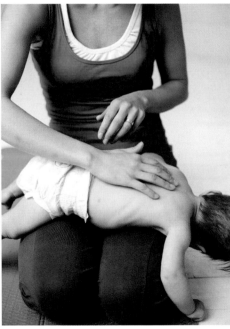 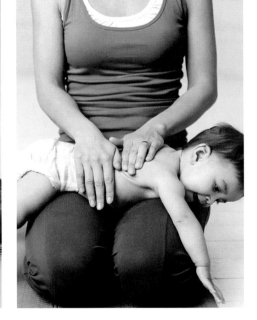

1 With alternate hands, keeping them soft, use your finger pads like cat paws to stroke your baby's back from the base of his neck all the way down to his lower back. Make sure that you keep continuous contact, with one hand on his back at all times. Avoid any pressure on his spine, stroking down on either side of it. Repeat three times with both hands.

2 Hands flat, use both together across your baby's upper back. Rub back and forth in opposite directions, going down the back to the buttocks and then back up to the shoulders. Repeat three times, adjusting the pressure to your baby's liking. Some babies enjoy far more pressure than you might have imagined was suitable.

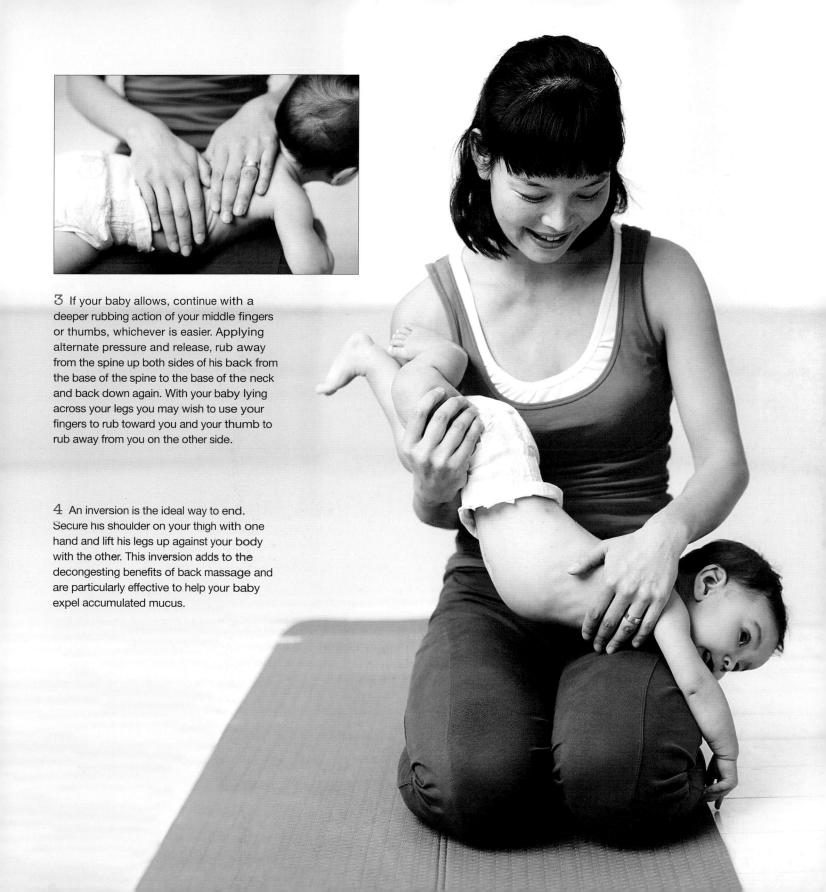

3 If your baby allows, continue with a deeper rubbing action of your middle fingers or thumbs, whichever is easier. Applying alternate pressure and release, rub away from the spine up both sides of his back from the base of the spine to the base of the neck and back down again. With your baby lying across your legs you may wish to use your fingers to rub toward you and your thumb to rub away from you on the other side.

4 An inversion is the ideal way to end. Secure his shoulder on your thigh with one hand and lift his legs up against your body with the other. This inversion adds to the decongesting benefits of back massage and are particularly effective to help your baby expel accumulated mucus.

Massaging his front

If your baby dislikes lying still on his back, stroke him whenever the opportunities arise—as you are dressing or undressing him, before or after his bath, or after changing his nappy. When he shows his enjoyment of these short practices, he may be ready to relax on his back again for an integrated massage with oil.

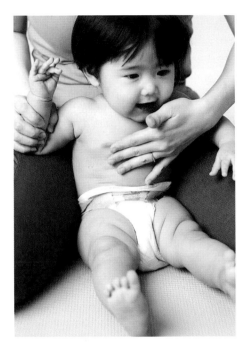

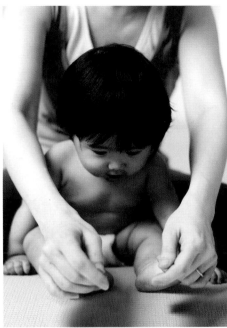

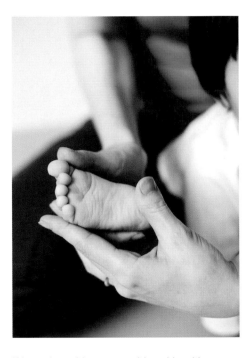

1 With your baby sitting in front of you, facing away, try a chest rub. Using the flat of your middle three fingers, rub in a circle from the center of his chest out to the side around his nipple and back. Repeat three times, adjusting your pressure. Using your other hand, do the same on the opposite side. You can use the rhyme: "Round and round the garden, like a teddy bear, round and round the garden, tickly under there."

2 Glide your hands along his legs to reach his feet, rather than suddenly grabbing one of them, and gently knead them, using your thumbs to apply and release pressure.

If he enjoys this, support his ankle with one hand and use your thumb to massage his feet (pages 24–25.) You can use the rhyme: "This little piggy went to market, this little piggy stayed at home. This little piggy had a massage, this little piggy had none, and this little piggy went whee whee whee all the way home."

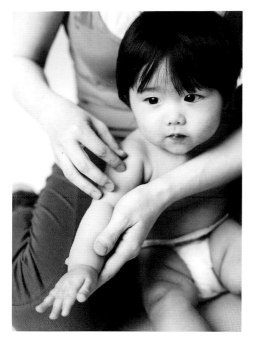

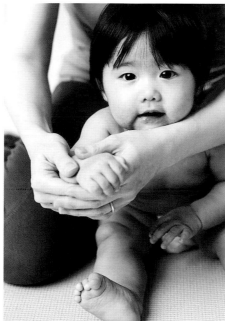

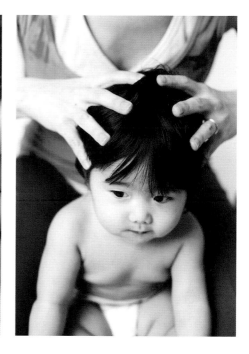

3 Make cat paws with your fingers to stroke your baby's arm down and up while supporting his wrist by bringing your other arm across his front.

If he enjoys this, alternately massage the palm and top of his hand with your thumb. Then roll each finger, either from the top or the palm, starting with the thumb. An appropriate rhyme is: "Tommy thumb, Tommy thumb, where are you? Here I am, Here I am, How do you do?" The fingers could be Peter Pointer, Toby Tall, Ruby Ring, and Baby Small.

4 Many babies welcome a head rub, particularly when they are sleepy. Use both hands to make small circular movements from front to back across his scalp with the pads of your fingers. Adjust the pressure to his liking, massaging the whole of his head down toward the back of his ears. Avoid pressing the fontanelles with your index fingers if they are still not fully closed.

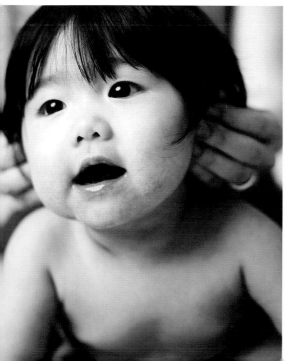

5 Continue by using your thumbs and middle fingers to rub his ears slowly and gently from top to lobe. Apply and release pressure along the rims of his ears, and roll the lobes between your thumbs and fingers. There are many nerve endings in the ear lobes and massage may be soothing if his molars are coming through.

Dynamic high lift and swing

Once you are able confidently to pick up your baby with a lift (as on page 109), turn it into a dynamic practice. Most babies find high lifts exciting but avoid them in the evenings when you are encouraging your baby to wind down, and also when he is quiet. As all baby yoga movements, high lifts and swings are best done in response to your baby's invite, in this case when he feels greater attraction to acrobatic moves.

High lift

From a semi-squat, take a deep breath and lift your baby, extending your legs and arms to the full. Raise him in one single movement without leaning back. Exhale and lower him to stand on the floor. To start with, have your baby facing you and once you have both grown in confidence, try lifting him facing away from you.

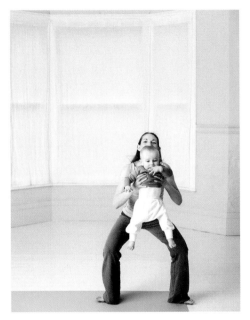
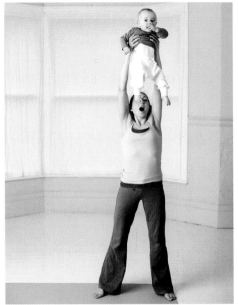

High swing

Join your hands across your baby's chest and lift him from the floor. Swing him gently at first, gathering momentum to swing him progressively higher to both sides of your body. Once you get into a steady rhythm, this high swing may be less demanding for you than a more restricted movement. Swing your baby to the rhythm of your breathing. Reduce the swinging span slowly to stop, and lower him gently, to protect your back.

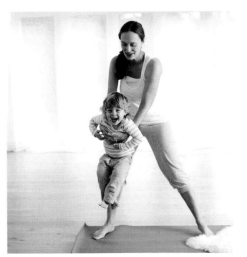
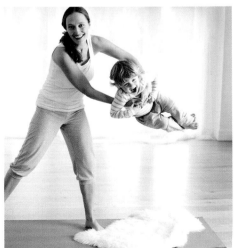

Imitation—how your baby learns

Your baby has been watching you since the day he was born. At first, his focus was on your face, but since the second half of his first year he has been registering your movements and, once mobile, he will actively attempt to copy them. The more you practice baby yoga with him, the more attentive he will become and the greater his anticipation actions in routine sequences. Your baby will be filled with delight at the knowledge that you have understood what he is trying to do. From that moment onward, your shared yoga practice becomes a game of imitation in which your baby registers more and more precisely what you are doing and then, often hours or even days later rather than instantly, enacts what he has observed.

Rather than praising your baby lavishly when he does this, show him your full version of the posture. Encouraging him to "perform" to an audience, or to camera, is not desirable at this stage because it curtails his genuine exploration of his body and range of movement. It is more helpful for him to watch you demonstrate the practice.

It may take a long time for your baby to extend his arms above his head from his first attempts at copying your stretch.

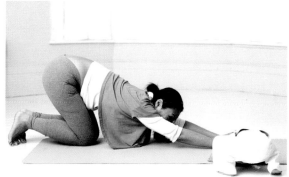

Pause now and again to notice that your baby's antics may actually reproduce some of your postnatal yoga stretches.

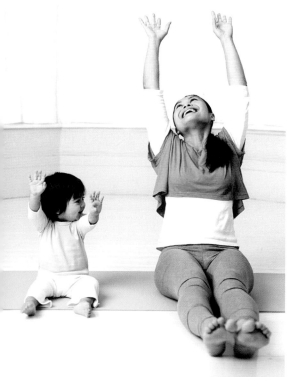

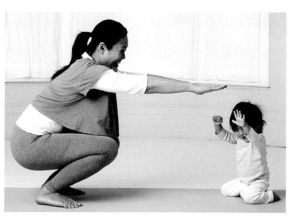

Babies may be able to reproduce one aspect of the practice they imitate and not others—a combination of squatting and forward arm extension is too demanding until much later on.

Secure standing to secure walking

Your baby's first independent step is a magical moment. It takes place against the invisible scaffolding made of all the practices that have helped to secure his standing and consolidate his balance to the point when he can finally accomplish the extraordinary feat of displacing his weight from one leg to the other while moving forward. In between standing and walking,

baby yoga can help to steady balance and reduce the occurrence of falls that may upset your baby. Better than any baby walker, your body offers a live support for your baby to test his standing balance and gain both steadiness and agility. Rather than encouraging your baby to walk, take time to enjoy this process while playing constructive games.

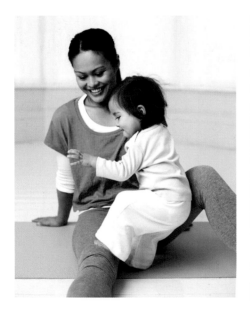

Stepping

Sit with your baby standing sideways between your legs. Bring one knee up to support his back while keeping your other leg extended. With or without the incentive of reaching for a toy, your baby will be interested in stepping over your leg. Be ready to give him a helping hand but try not to interfere until it proves necessary.

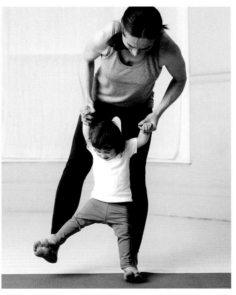

Giant steps

Place your baby's feet on top of yours and immediately start walking with her, holding her wrists loosely enough for her to find her own balance. The more you raise your legs, the more challenging this game becomes.

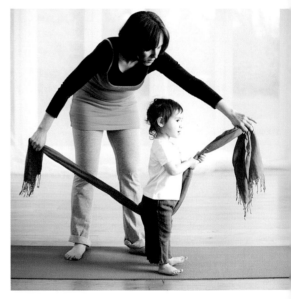

Soft horse

Place a long scarf between your baby's legs and hold it at the front and back so that she can ride this imaginary horse. Support under her seat may be just what she needs to gain further stability in stepping forward or sideways. A soft horse encourages further bouncing on one spot, which may be necessary to top up leg strength before walking feels possible.

Leg lift duo

If you do yoga balances on one leg, your baby may be keen to try daring standing balances with hand support from you. In any case, try some leg lifts to promote his balance and alignment.

Lean him forward while holding his hands and stretching his arms up and wide. This gives him a solid base to raise his back leg.

Holding your baby's arm and leg on one side gives him a head start for securely balancing on one foot. Make sure you do this on both sides.

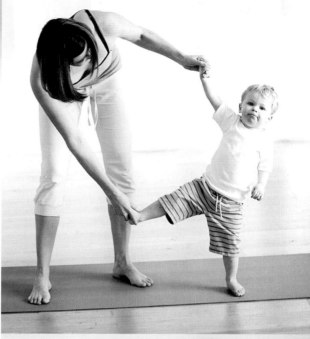

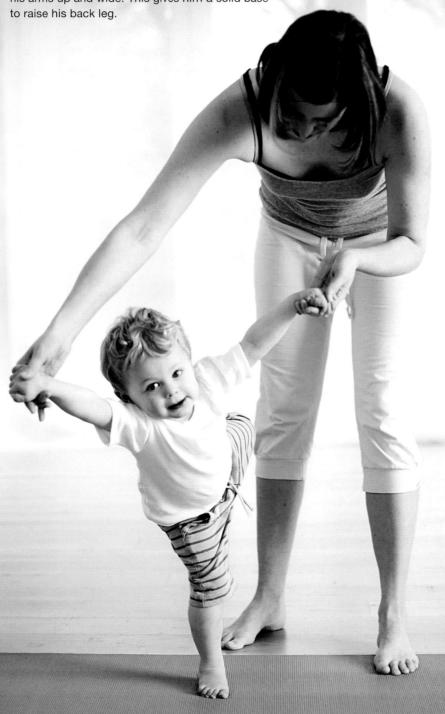

Walk with a goose step, which your baby may be inspired to join in. With practice, he will be able to hold his leg up for a few seconds while you breathe through this yoga pose and tone your abdominals.

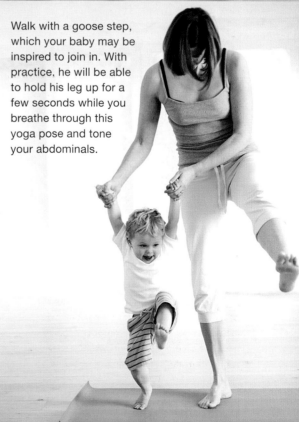

Kneeling flow inversion

Your baby may now be too tall and too heavy for you to practice inversions in a sitting position. Kneeling is a safe and more comfortable base from which to add new turns, against the support of your body. Lifting your baby upside down securely from his hips at first, rather than attempting to hold him from his feet, ensures greater protection for his head and neck in the landing phase. The following sequence, just slightly modified since earlier inversions, will give him a sense of continuity in the midst of change. With experience, you will be able to integrate the steps into a smooth, flowing movement, flipping your baby upside down and back to his feet again with the safe support of your body in between.

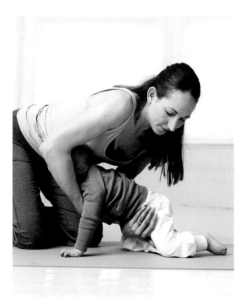

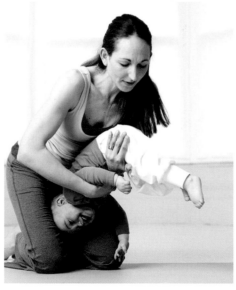

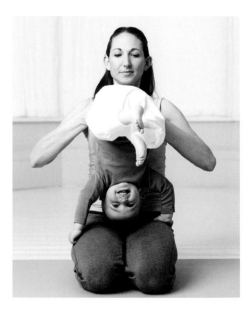

1 Pick up your baby, whether he is on all fours or standing, supporting him under his hips and upper chest.

2 Take a breath and swivel him head down against your body as you sit up on your knees. His head is resting softly on your lap, between your thighs.

3 Exhale and bring your baby's back to rest against the front of your body as you steady yourself in a vertical position, sitting on your heels. If your baby is very tall or your arms ache, come up to a kneeling position with your back fully extended. Whichever position you choose, you need to place your hands securely on your baby's hips first, as the length of his back stretches against your stomach and chest.

4 Take a breath and, with a secure hip hold, lift your baby, raising your arms or raising your seat from your heels, or both at once. Practice this in front of a mirror to see his reaction. Hold for no more than four seconds. Then lower him right against your body with his legs to either side of your head, so that his shoulders rest on the base of your rib cage. Lean back a little to take his legs over in front of you while lowering him toward your thighs. He will simultaneously right himself to face you.

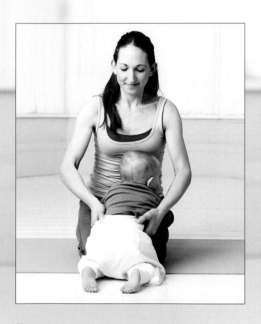

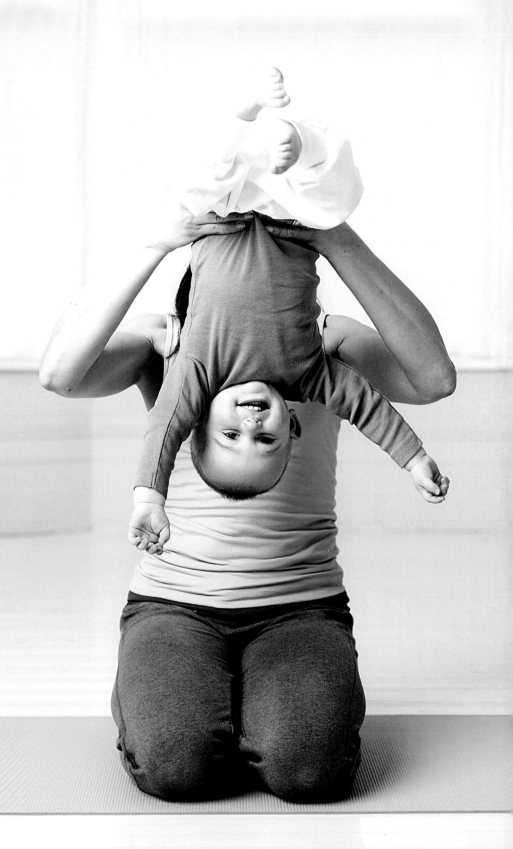

5 Once your baby has landed, on an all-fours or in a standing position, allow him to find his bearings before you repeat the practice. Twice is sufficient, even if he asks for more.

First handstand

Handstands help babies to develop arm and back strength in just the same way as they are used in classic yoga. Once you see your baby pressing his hands onto the floor in an upside-down pose he can hold for up to a minute if undisturbed, it is time to try handstands. In order to help him get the greatest benefit from the practice, what matters most is how you handle his hips and lower back. If you follow the instructions below carefully, you can then lift your baby upside down directly from a handstand in a way that supports his alignment and feels gentle and safe to him.

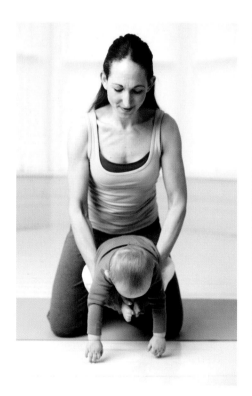 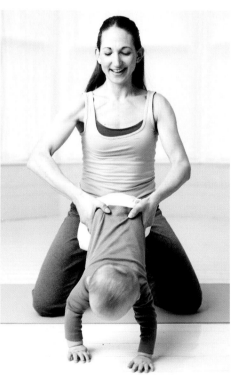 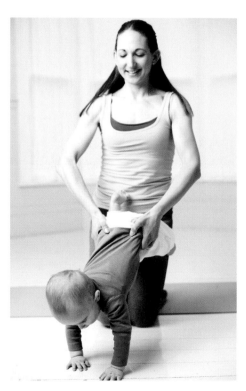

1 Test your baby's readiness by allowing him to lean forward from butterfly hold, while raising yourself from sitting on your heels to a high kneeling position.

2 If your baby is ready for handstands, he may start walking his hands away from you. You can alternately raise his hips and lower his bent legs in order to help him gain greater lower back strength.

3 As he gains strength and pushes himself into a more upright posture, you will need to raise yourself even higher on your knees. Keep pivoting his hips and taking his legs under his hips so that he can land in a kneeling position or a squat rather than falling flat on his upper chest when his arms give in and bend.

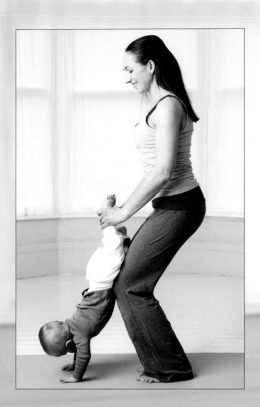

4 When his arms are pushing strongly from the floor, slide your hands along his legs to complete his handstand. You will have to get up in order to support his hips against your bent knees. Step back and bring his legs under his body rather than allowing him to collapse.

5 If you feel strong enough, lift your baby off the ground, resting his chest and hips on your bent legs to ensure an optimal spinal stretch. Lower him gently, allowing him to go back to a handstand before stepping back and bringing his legs under his body for a safe landing.

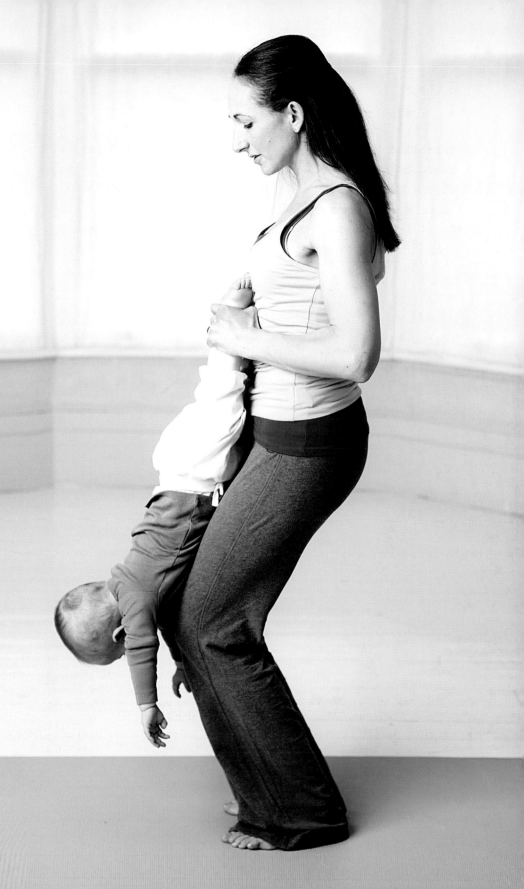

Roly-polies

If your baby likes to go upside down and press his head on the floor, he may be ready for supported roly-polies. While he is trying to push his bottom up, you can take hold of his hips and guide him through the aligned moves that will ensure a predictable roll. The streamlined action will enhance his body awareness and give him a sense of future economy of movement and effective use of all his muscles. Inevitably, this will also result in greater body confidence and agility, boosting his overall self-confidence. Sideways rolls are another enjoyable challenge. Show him what to do and he will discover the spinal moves for himself.

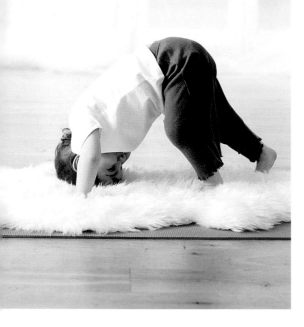

When you see your baby practicing a head-down dog pose, the time may be right for a roly-poly.

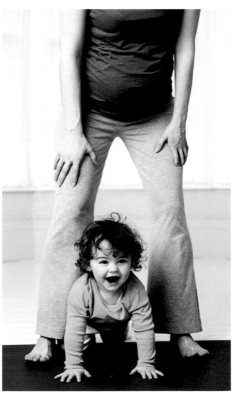

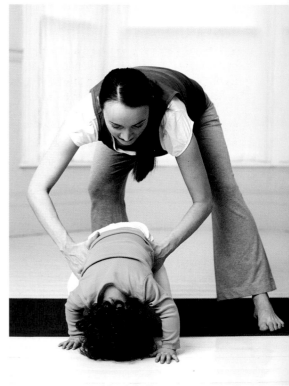

Test his readiness by taking a secure hold of his hips when he is on all fours, and lifting his bent legs up gently. He may try a handstand, pushing with his hands to lift his head, or he may leave head and hands on the floor with his bottom up in the air as you support his weight from the hips. Respect his choice.

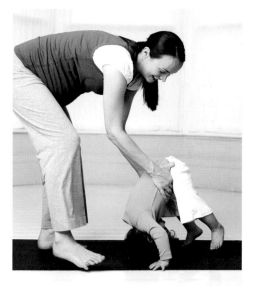 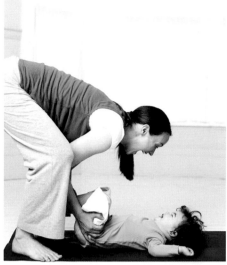 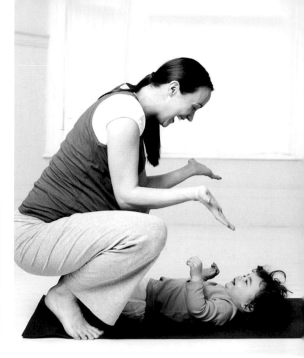

1 For greater ease and safe execution of this move, stand facing your baby's back as he puts his head down on the floor. Announce you are about to join in by saying "Ready, go!" Gently but firmly take hold of his hips and bring them up and forward to ensure a safe, soft roll, protecting his neck.

2 There may be an instant of surprise as your baby finds himself on his back, facing you.

3 This will not be the last time he is taken unawares as he starts taking risks. In baby yoga, you strike a delicate balance between supporting your child in moves that he shows you he is ready to complete and reassuring him that, well, life is full of surprises!

Sideways roll

It seems a long time since your baby launched himself in his first roll from lying on his back to being on his front or vice versa. As he gained back strength and mobility, he was able to change position without rolling. Now his development takes him back to the exploration of rolling, this time as a continuous movement— enjoyable but challenging to execute at first. Modeling sideways rolls for your baby is the best way for you to guide him into independent rolling.

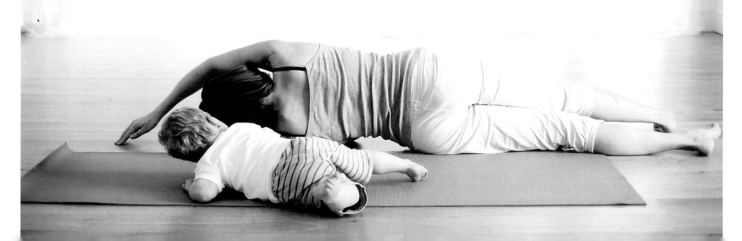

Balances for walking babies and toddlers

Show your baby how to walk along a scarf or belt, placing one foot in front of the other, and then watch her do it by herself. This exercise will help her balance and increase her confidence. Most toddlers enjoy negotiating circuits with specific obstacles and challenges to overcome along the way.

Lie a long scarf on your yoga mat and let your baby follow you along it. At first she may step across the scarf to create an easier challenge for herself, or even trample it in frustration. Gradually, she will discover the use of her arms and be able to walk along a narrow belt with a visible sense of mastery.

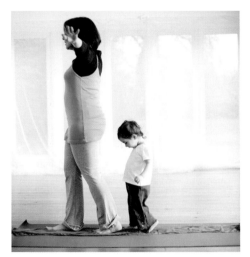 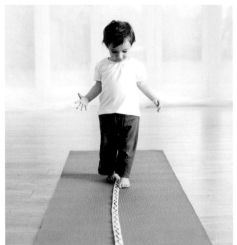

Your baby may find it difficult at first to get up or down a step on her feet, and foam blocks can help. Up is easier than down, and she is likely to bring both feet onto the block. Eventually, she will be able to step up with one foot and then down on the other side with the other foot in one movement. This will give her a secure foundation to approach stairs later on.

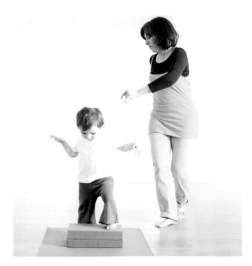 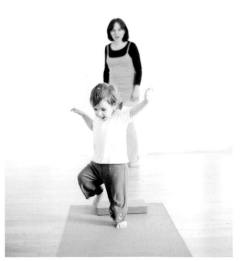

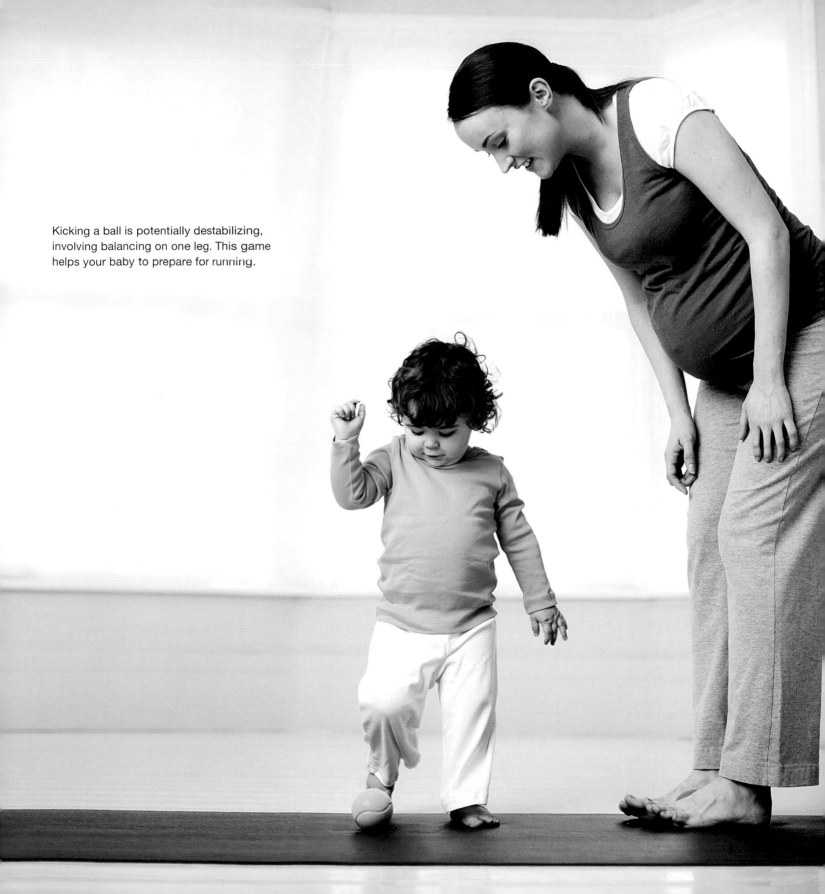

Kicking a ball is potentially destabilizing, involving balancing on one leg. This game helps your baby to prepare for running.

Jolly jumpers

Jumping is an accomplishment that many babies do not acquire until their third year. From early in their second year, they start preparing themselves for taking off from the floor but this may not be immediately visible. Watch for early signs and encourage your toddler to hop and skip until he is ready to keep his feet together. Hop, skip, and jump through the day whenever a need arises for a short energetic practice.

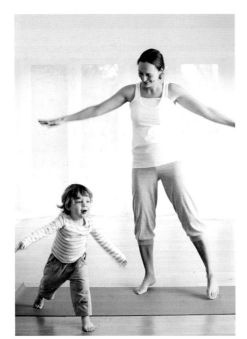

Starting with the flying arm movement of a bird or a jet plane, according to your toddler's imagery, encourage him to lift one leg off the floor, then the other.

Watch him discover the alternate movement of his arms that naturally accompanies skipping, as he finds that he can hop to shift his weight. This can be a very exciting turning point in your toddler's development.

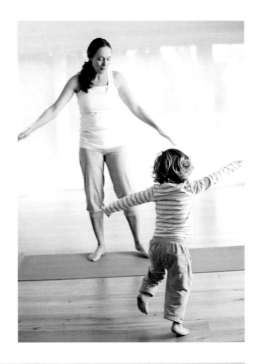

Your toddler may now stand steadily on a foam block but still step down from it rather than jump off it with his two feet together. A light support with a rhythmical action can help make the transition to jumping an easy and fun one.

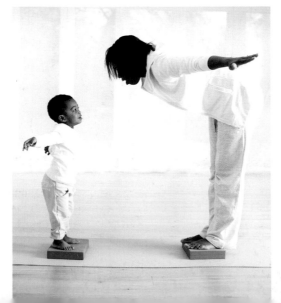

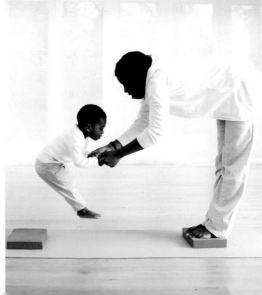

Circular walking relaxation

Many toddlers try to soothe themselves by walking in circles, often counterclockwise. Inadvertently, as they go faster and faster this may trigger more excitement than soothing. Slow down your toddler with a rhythmical, circular walk of your own. Use this circular walking often, after an upset, a separation, or when your baby suddenly starts waking up in the night for no obvious reason.

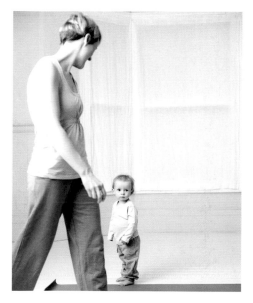 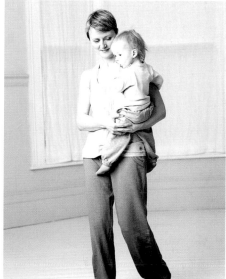

When your baby starts walking in a circle, you do the same. Carry him when he gets tired or upset. It is best not to talk but rather to concentrate on the rhythm of your breathing and your steps. Concentrate on walking the circle with your baby in your arms, and deepen your relaxation as you exhale with each alternate step. Now and again, stop to give him a gentle kiss and reassure him. This deepens his relaxed state and consequently yours, too.

Beneficial effects

With practice, your calm breathing and walking rhythms will become so familiar that they will act as a signal to your toddler, and induce a relaxation response. This will help him settle with less distress than might otherwise be the case, and has beneficial effects on his nervous system at a time when his brain is still rapidly developing. You can also use circular walking as a preparation for lying-down relaxation. Your mobile baby may not be prepared to lie down too, but being aware that you are relaxing will help him understand that relaxation is integral to yoga and an essential completion of the fun stretchy part.

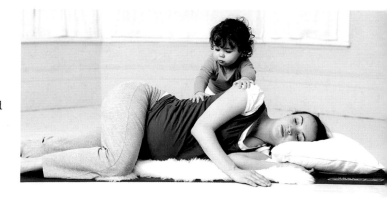

Your relaxation helps toddlers resolve extreme emotions. Tolerate tugs, slaps, and kisses, remaining neutral, even though at other times setting boundaries has priority.

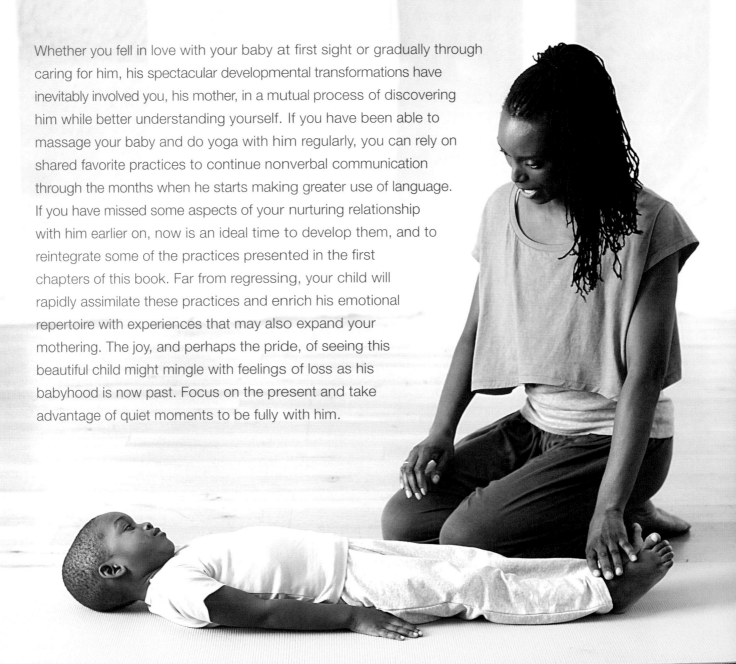

7 Toddler Yoga

Whether you fell in love with your baby at first sight or gradually through caring for him, his spectacular developmental transformations have inevitably involved you, his mother, in a mutual process of discovering him while better understanding yourself. If you have been able to massage your baby and do yoga with him regularly, you can rely on shared favorite practices to continue nonverbal communication through the months when he starts making greater use of language. If you have missed some aspects of your nurturing relationship with him earlier on, now is an ideal time to develop them, and to reintegrate some of the practices presented in the first chapters of this book. Far from regressing, your child will rapidly assimilate these practices and enrich his emotional repertoire with experiences that may also expand your mothering. The joy, and perhaps the pride, of seeing this beautiful child might mingle with feelings of loss as his babyhood is now past. Focus on the present and take advantage of quiet moments to be fully with him.

Hip sequence with back arch

Manually guiding your toddler in stretches is still the best way of revisiting earlier poses. Most two year olds enjoy being on their backs after mastering mobility skills. Start with the supine hip sequence, introducing different angles and moves better suited to a toddler than a baby. Afterward, align his legs and feet for a lying-down relaxation, which you can introduce with a few long massage strokes from head to toes.

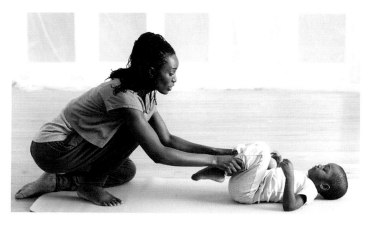

1 Knees to chest still helps digestion and to combat constipation. Take his bent knees as far up his body as possible, applying firm downward pressure, and then extend his legs back toward you. Encourage him to inhale as his legs are extended and exhale deeply when his knees are being pressed down. If his head is not flat on the mat, place a small cushion under it.

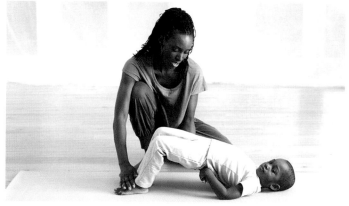

2 Low bridge pose, a lower back strengthener, is the counterpose to knees to chest. Help your child raise his tailbone higher by pressing his feet to the mat with one hand and extending your other arm under the back of his waist for additional support.

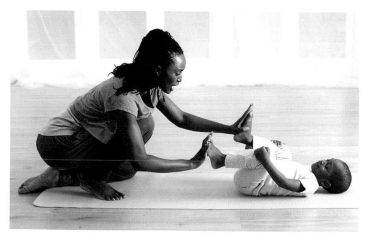

3 To relax and tone his back after low bridge pose, modify push-counterpush (pages 54–55) by pressing against his feet horizontally rather than from above. By now, he can offer substantial resistance and, if he chooses to push hard, you may need all your arm strength in order to move his legs like pistons. The greater his resistance, the better this practice works as a back toner.

Hip sequence with handstand

Yoga with toddlers, as a means of communication through touch and movement, requires getting ready together. Before you start a practice, make time to listen to your child, harmonize your moods and, if you are about to do something new with him, talk about it first.

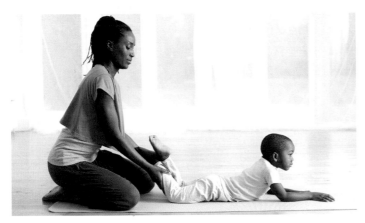

1 Mini cobra

The stretch that helped your baby gain strength to lift his head now prepares your toddler for handstand. Start with a stretch on forearms rather than on hands for a progressive action on the middle spine, and guide him to deepen his breathing, pressing on his forearms as he exhales.

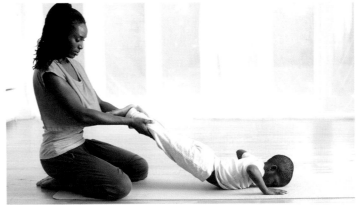

2 Leg lift

Start by raising his legs gently as he lies on his front with his arms and head relaxed on the mat. Encourage him to breathe deeper to keep his legs up. Hold his feet again, higher this time, and ask him to place his hands to the sides of his neck and press them on the floor through three deep breaths, to strengthen his lumbar spine.

3 Handstand

Ask him to press harder on his hands and to make his back strong as you kneel up to raise his legs. If his ribcage collapses forward because his mid-back and abdominal muscles are not yet strong enough, lower his legs slowly.

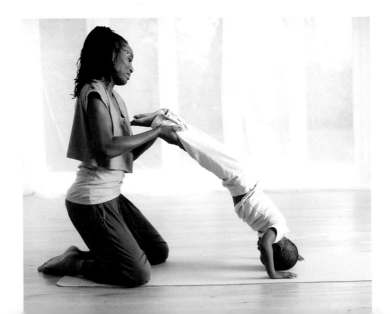

Introducing classic yoga postures

Your child is now starting to extend his legs and arms fully, but will still need the support of your body to move on to the classic poses. You can help him to align his spine and adjust the position of his feet, head, and arms. Here are a few examples among the many postures you can practice together.

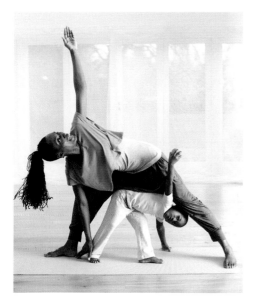

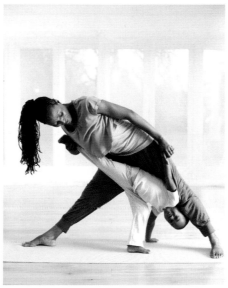

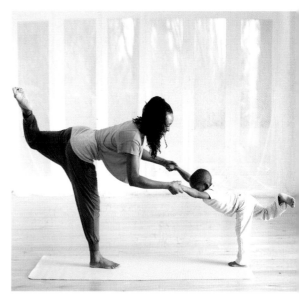

1 Triangle pose
Having your child back to front against your body allows you to stabilize his back foot with one hand. While maintaining your pose, use your other hand to help him align his top hip and shoulder and gently stretch his arm back. With time, his front leg will straighten in a classic triangle pose.

2 Moon pose
From a triangle leg base (his and yours), raise his back leg while supporting him against your body and back leg. Experiencing the alignment of a pose will help him to understand later adjustments.

3 Warrior balance
Hold his hands to stabilize him. It will be some time before he can fully extend his back leg but his stance and balance will improve month by month.

Yoga together

Yoga practice with friends is fun and stimulating for both toddlers and adults. Joint yoga provides an opportunity to try partner exercises that give toddlers a sense of harmony and integration, and a space for noncompetitive interaction between parents and children, in which different skills and achievements can be celebrated. Partner poses that toddlers can do together make yoga easier and more beneficial for them, and may also facilitate the transition from yoga with mother to independent yoga.

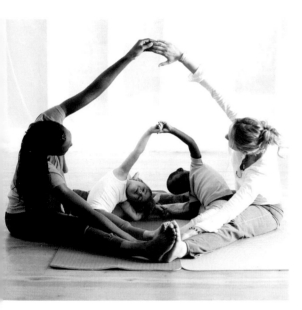

Heart opener

Toddlers still enjoy being contained in a safe space. Stretching together in parallel with mothers whose extended legs make a diamond enclosure in a sitting position is peaceful and comforting. Breathing rhythms can be taught with the slow flow of this side stretch that also opens the heart area.

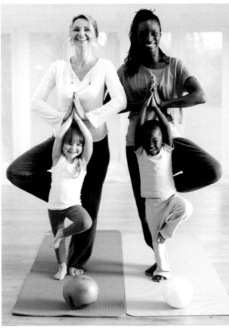

Tree pose

Hold your toddler's hands between your hands as she stands in front of you. Your toddler may already be able to balance on one leg but the support of your body allows her to stretch her arms up. Together with friends, the relaxation that this most ancient pose can bring is felt more easily.

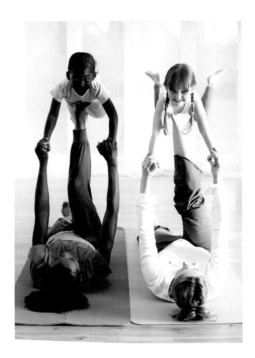

Foot balance

You can lift your toddler safely by placing your foot against her sternum, in the center of her chest. Gradually extend your leg while holding her hands, bending it again to bring her back to standing if the pose feels unstable at any time. If you are both stable and comfortable, you can bring your other foot under your child's chest for a fuller stretch of both your legs. Doing this with a friend is more thrilling than any fun fair!

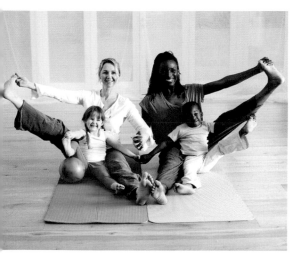

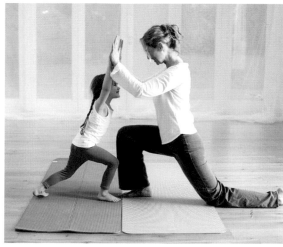

Leg stretch and warrior pose together

Holding hands in the middle makes it easier for two mothers sitting side by side with their toddlers to do a leg stretch while remaining aligned. Repeat on the other side, and complement this pose with a warrior pose with your toddler.

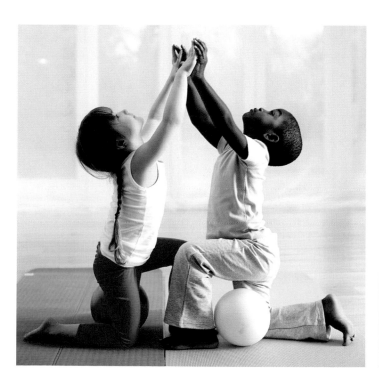

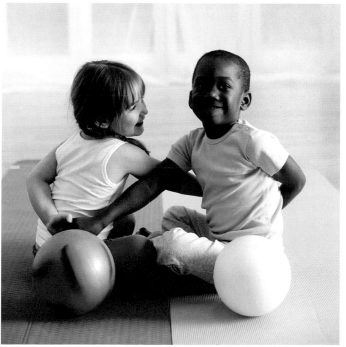

Half kneeling stretch together

Sitting on a ball may stabilize your toddler in half-kneeling poses. By pressing the palms of their hands together, toddlers can help each other stretch up to an extent that they could not achieve singly. Repeat on the other side.

Sitting pretzel

Continue with a sitting twist making the shape of a pretzel. Prepare by crossing hands, then flexing and extending arms alternately to the rhythm of the breath. Then ask both toddlers to extend the arm they have been using behind their back. Reaching for their friend's hand with their free hand, they then pull each other in a classic yoga twist. Repeat on the other side.

Story time

Toddlers' imaginations are developing rapidly and they love simple stories in which they can impersonate animals and elements. Besides promoting spinal alignment, balance, and flexibility, yoga also helps toddlers give physical expression to emotions, images, and even adventures. Rather than imposing and correcting classic yoga poses inspired by animals, the priority is to allow toddlers to express their feelings, prompted by stories and their own perception of animals.

Bunnies help the sun rise

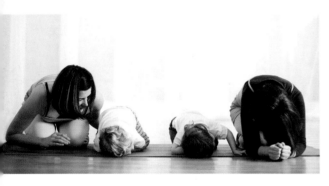

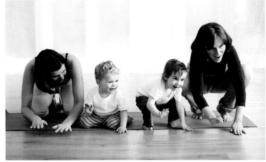

1 Start your story with bunnies in a deep sleep, and encourage the toddlers to be very still, kneeling with heads on the mat. Speak slowly and dramatically, lengthening vowels: "Bunnies are faaast asleep in the daark night …"

2 "Bunnies are woken up by a light. They take a peep out of their little houses to see what's happening. Shush, be quiet, let's find out. Go through the rabbit hole slowly, without making any noise …"

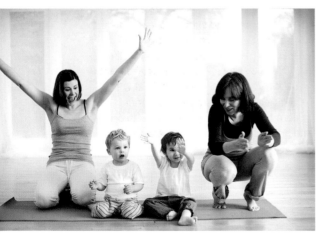

3 "Sit on the hill! Look! The big orange sun has just appeared far away across the fields. It is sooo huge! We bunnies can help the sun rise with our hops and jumps, let's go and help the sun rise …"

4 "Stretch up to the sky, open your arms wide and stretch up more. The sun is rising fast, bunnies can dance and be merry all day."

Other animals join in

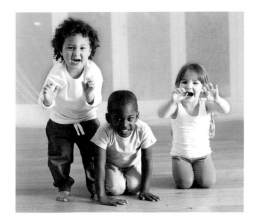

A fox appears … an impersonation of a fox helps this three year old to integrate earlier yoga stretches he has experienced into an impressive commando crawl. Watch out bunnies!

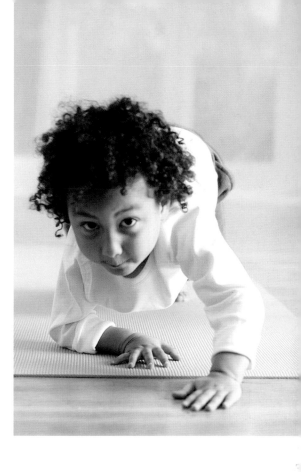

Bunnies become lions … seeing lions, bunnies do tremendous hops to escape. But bunnies ARE the lions! They tense their bodies and make claws to impersonate fierceness. Khiani in the middle does not want to be a harmful animal and decides to be a cat.

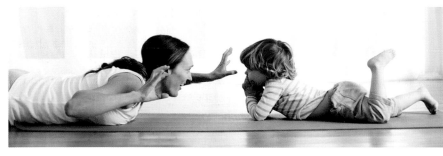

Watch out for lion-crocodiles … in the meantime, down by the river, mother has seen a crocodile and shows how wide he can snap. Alvar remembers the rhyme "Row, row, row your boat, gently down the stream, if you see a crocodile, don't forget to scream," which he has practiced with his mother in baby yoga. His idea of a scream to ward off crocodiles colludes with his most terrifying lion impersonation.

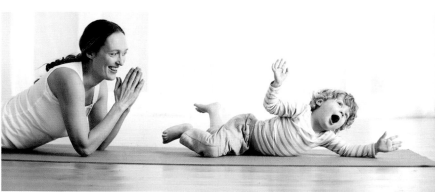

Relaxation with toddlers

As your toddler increasingly asserts himself in his quest for independence, and the "terrible twos" challenge you to the limit of your patience and understanding, sharing moments of relaxation is crucial. Toddlers often welcome and appreciate massage because it provides continuity with earlier times. Besides completing every yoga practice, relaxation techniques provide a structured way for you and your child to return to calm and harmony after confrontations and allow loving feelings to resurface. You can use these techniques whenever the need arises. By giving your toddler body-based resources to calm down, center himself, and restore peace, you are equipping him with invaluable life skills.

Containing hold, resolution, and relaxation

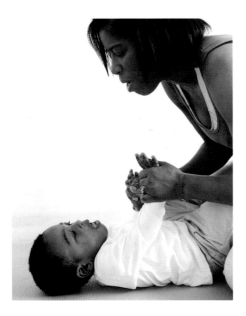 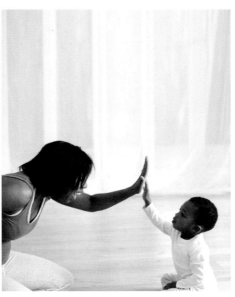 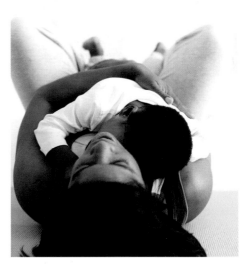

After a temper tantrum, a containing hold may still help your toddler to get out of his distress bubble and back to the here and now, just as containment helped him as a tiny baby. Make sure that your hold is firm and loving, free from anger. Calm yourself, as well as calming him, by slowing your breathing. If he is still screaming, you can say, "It's OK now," on each exhalation.

Actively expressing resolution is positive for a toddler. A high five can be used in many different ways to release pent-up energy, express residual aggression in a playful way, and mostly to make friendly contact through your joint palms.

Toddlers are often exhausted after confrontations with their parents. This is when they feel the need for a loving hug and welcome close relaxation on your body in a way you could not have imagined a moment earlier. Take this opportunity to relax deeply and to acknowledge the loving bond between you and your child.

Blowing bubbles

Hand massage and a song

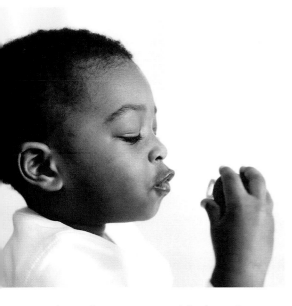
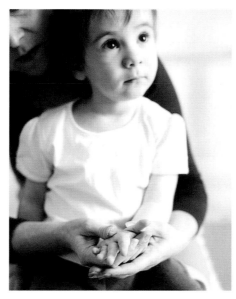
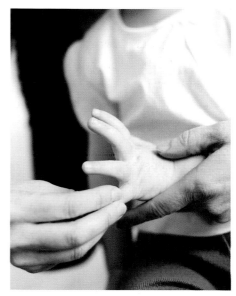

In a calm state, your toddler is ready for expanding his breath awareness. Blowing bubbles can help him lengthen his exhalation the yoga way, to make optimal use of his lung capacity. Long exhalations help draw oxygenated air to the back of the lungs more efficiently than increasing intake of air with forceful inspirations.

If time is short, or you are not in a suitable place for lying-down relaxation, remember that hand massage can be instantly soothing for your toddler. Start with the left hand. Circular rubbing of her palm with your thumb is particularly effective, from the inner wrist to the center. While massaging her fingers you can remind her of the baby finger rhymes you may have sung to her earlier on. The combination of hand massage and singing helps release oxytocin, the love hormone, in both your and her bloodstream. This is cumulative and each practice adds to the previous one.

Your relaxation matters

Short relaxations can create mini-rhythms in your day with a toddler. This will help you refresh yourself at regular intervals in a way that your toddler acknowledges and learns to respect. Integrating relaxation in flexible yet stabilizing forms brings yoga to the core of our lives. In harmony with the ancient principles of yoga and the other traditions that have inspired this book, by nurturing yourself, you can best nurture your whole family.

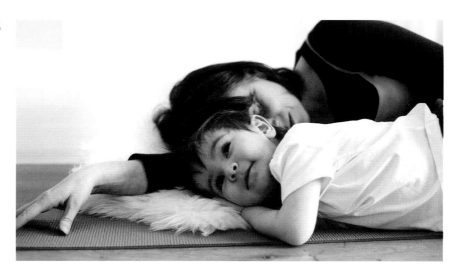

Sun salutation

Performed with flowing movement, and attention to the breath, the salute to the sun stimulates the whole body in two to three minutes. From the age of three, small children are able to memorize the sequence, and early practice develops strength, flexibility, and coordination. Done with a friend, it promotes synchronization in a noncompetitive spirit. Here are simple teaching points for you to guide the children.

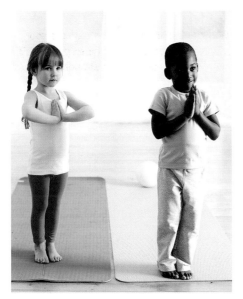

1 Prayer pose. Stand up straight and try to keep your feet together. Join your hands, palms together, in front of your heart. Feel strong and quiet at the same time.

2 Big stretch up. Extend your arms forward and lift them up above your head with one great breath. Keep your feet together if you can while you stretch up.

The next move is head to knees, as in Step 7: blow out while bending forward with your legs straight. Look at your knees and put your hands or fingers on the floor on each side of your feet if you can reach.

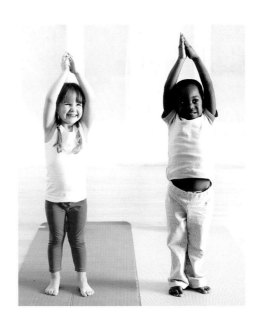

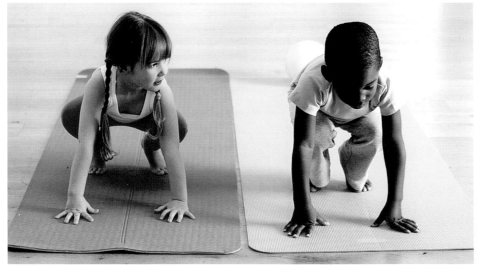

3 Backward lunge. Keeping your hands on the floor, prepare for a backward lunge (opposite of forward lunge, Step 6). Take a breath, bend one leg and extend the other back behind you. It is fine to have the knee of your back leg on the floor.

Move from there into a down dog, as in Step 5. Pushing from your hands on the floor, extend your front foot back to join your back foot. Lift your hips high and try to straighten your arms and legs, push and breathe strongly.

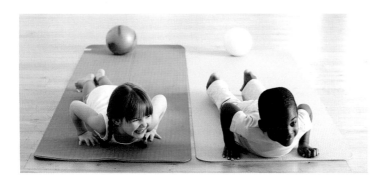

4 Eight-limb crawl. Keep your hands in the same position as in down dog and come down on your knees. Then bring your chest, and, if you can, also your chin to the floor.

Then move into the cobra. Slide forward onto your tummy and press on your hands with your bent arms to lift your shoulders and chest up. Breathe strongly in this cobra pose.

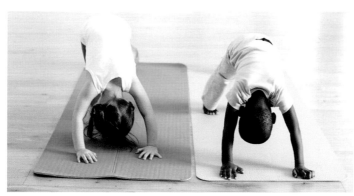

5 Down dog. Push from your hands on the floor, tuck your toes under and lift your hips up in the air again in down dog pose. Breathe strongly.

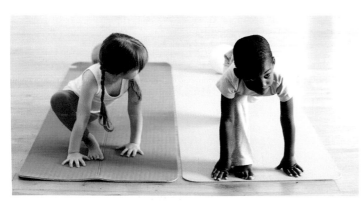

6 Forward lunge. Take a breath and step one of your feet forward between your hands. Drop your back knee to the floor in this lunge and look up if you can.

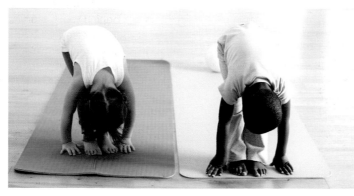

7 Head to knees. Blow out while bending forward with your legs straight. Look at your knees and put your hands or fingers on the floor on each side of your feet if you can reach.

Then extend your arms forward and lift them up above your head with one great breath. Keep your feet together if you can while you stretch up as in Step 2. To end, and start a new round, return to the prayer pose, Step 1. For three year olds, two rounds is enough.

Index

Resources

Current Birthlight centers and partner centers worldwide

Birthlight UK
www.birthlight.com

Birthlight Center Zurich
www.birthlight.ch

Birthlight New Zealand
www.essentialmidwife.co.uk

Birthlight Institute Singapore
www.inspiremumbaby.com

Birthlight Germany
www.birthlight.de

Birthlight Taiwan
www.in-mommy.com

Birthlight Center Moscow
www.birthlight.ru

Birthlight Holland
www.yogamoves.nl

Birthlight Hungary
www.jogaszules.info

Acknowledgments

Author's acknowledgments

I would like to thanks Sally Lomas, as the Birthlight tutor who has most contributed to promote Birthlight Baby Yoga, together with tutors Melanie Hamilton Davies and Liz Doherty. Thanks to Jay Ehrlich for making this book possible and for her dedication to yoga with special babies. Thanks to Ingrid Lewis and Kirsteen Ruffell for an inspiring photo shoot in London, Ian Boddy for making babies' subtle moves beautifully visible, and the whole CICO team for co-creating the joy of this book.

Publisher's acknowledgments

With many thanks to our models: Nancy and Lola; Vimmi, Roshan, and Raj; Angus, Conor, and Rohan; Anna and Juliet; Nadia and Freya; Susan and Oscar; Dean, Emma, and Daisy; Philippa and Ines; Akiko and Ellie; Kathryn and Xavier; Tabitha and Sian; Helen and Romy; Naoko and Eiji; Ricardo and Lola; Carmen and Lucas; Vedina and Skyla; Joanne and Charlotte; Nuri; Ariana and Syrifa; Emi and Nina; Freddie and Tillie; Jasper and Christy; Emma and Lois; Jay, Andy, and Jack; Kirsteen and Kali; Chloe, Ollie, and Pia; Julia and Rufus; Elisabeth, Alvar, and Clara; Alice and Millie; Bridget and August; Paulette, Morgan, and Ethan; Ori-Shemma and Khiani; Ingrid and Ineya; Natalie and Oscar; Helen and Amie.

Many thanks also to Marion and Jacqui for all their hard work and effort in bringing the book together and ensuring that everything ran smoothly.